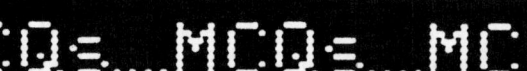

Paul Butler · Charles G. Blakeney
Alan Brooks · Robert Speller

FRCR Part I

Springer-Verlag
London Berlin Heidelberg New York
Paris Tokyo Hong Kong

Paul Butler, MRCP, FRCR
Consultant Neuroradiologist, The Royal London Hospital, Whitechapel,
London E1 1BB, and Honorary Senior Lecturer,
The Royal Free Hospital, Pond Street, London NW3 2QG

Charles G. Blakeney, MA, FRCR
Consultant Radiologist, The Royal London Hospital, Whitechapel, London
E1 1BB

Alan Brooks, MB, BS, BSc, DMRD, FRCR
Senior Lecturer in Radiology and Honorary Consultant,
St Bartholomew's Hospital, West Smithfield, London EC1A 7BE, and
The Royal London Hospital, Whitechapel, London E1 1BB

Robert Speller, BSc, ARCS, DIC, PhD
Senior Lecturer, Head of Academic Radiation Physics,
University College London, Medical Physics Department, 11–20 Capper Street,
London WC1E 6JA

Publisher's note: The "Brainscan" logo is reproduced by courtesy of
The Editor, *Geriatric Medicine*, Modern Medicine GB Ltd.

British Library Cataloguing in Publication Data
FRCR part 1.
1. Medicine. Radiology   I. Butler, Paul *1952–*   II. Series   616.0757

Library of Congress Cataloging-in-Publication Data
FRCR Part 1/Paul Butler . . . [et al.].
p. cm.
". . . designed for radiologists studying for the Part 1 examination for the
Fellowship of the Royal College of Radiologists . . ."–Pref.

ISBN 978-3-540-19620-4   ISBN 978-1-4471-1791-9 (eBook)
DOI 10.1007/978-1-4471-1791-9

1. Radiography. Medical–Examinations, questions, etc. I. Butler, Paul.
1952 June 4–
RC78.15.F73 1991   616.07'57'076–dc20   90–49697 CIP

Typeset by Wilmaset, Birkenhead, Wirral

2128/3830–543210 Printed on acid-free paper

Preface

This book of multiple choice questions is designed for radiologists studying for the Part 1 examination for the fellowship of the Royal College of Radiologists of the United Kingdom (Part 1 FRCR) but it is hoped that it will prove useful for all those beginning their radiology training and for radiographers studying for a higher diploma. The questions are derived from those used in a successful Part 1 FRCR Revision Course held annually by the Departments of Radiology of The Royal London and St Bartholomew's Hospitals, London, UK.

The first year trainee radiologist has to be something of a polymath, acquiring a breadth of basic knowledge which his or her seniors, individually, will find hard to match. It is unfortunate but true that further training as a senior registrar and the focusing as consultant on his or her special interest will mean that a greater or lesser amount of the Part 1 syllabus will simply be forgotten. The authors, therefore, make no apology for their number and even then each of us has had to call upon the expertise of others. In particular we would like to thank Dr Neil Garvie, Consultant in Radiology and Nuclear Medicine, The Royal London Hospital, and Dr Julie A. Horrocks, Mr L. Loverock and Mr I. Cullum, each of University College and Middlesex Hospital School of Medicine. Dr S. McGee, Registrar in Radiology at The Royal London Hospital, kindly reviewed all of the questions and made valuable comments for which the authors are grateful. Miss Pethroma Carr typed much of the manuscript.

The five examinations are "self contained" and in the style of the Part 1 FRCR MCQ examinations. If the reader works assiduously through each he or she will cover a large proportion of the syllabus for the Part I FRCR.

The material has been drawn largely from the suggested reading list available from the Royal College of Radiologists of the United Kingdom and, where necessary, references are given with the answers. An additional source for many of the physics questions has been *A Handbook of Physics for Radiologists and Radiographers* by D. Gifford (published by John Wiley, 1984).

London
1990

Paul Butler
Charles G. Blakeney
Alan Brooks
Robert Speller

Contents

The time allowed for each examination is 3 hours.

The answer to each of the parts of a question is either "true" or "false". There is no restriction on the number of "true" or "false" answers to any question.

A correct answer scores $+1$ mark, an incorrect answer -1. An unanswered question scores 0.

Abbreviations

AP	anteroposterior
C	cervical
CT	computed tomography
DSA	digital subtraction angiography
FO	fronto-occipital
HU	Hounsfield Units
L	lumbar
LAO	left anterior oblique
MR(I)	magnetic resonance (imaging)
PA	posteroanterior
RAO	right anterior oblique
T	thoracic

Examination 1

Questions

Q.1.1 **The spectrum from a tungsten target x-ray tube**

a. consists of only continuous radiation when operated at 65 kVp
b. consists of only characteristic x-rays when operated at 80 kVp and above
c. depends upon the mA used
d. can be directly determined using an ionisation chamber
e. will change with distance from the x-ray tube

Q.1.2 **The apparent focal spot size of a rotating anode tube**

a. varies along the anode–cathode line
b. depends upon the distance between the filament and the anode
c. depends upon the diameter of the rotating anode disc
d. depends upon the filament current
e. depends upon the speed of anode rotation

Q.1.3 **In x-ray production the importance of the product kVp × mAs is that it is proportional to**

a. the effective energy of the x-ray beam
b. the total x-ray scatter
c. the heat produced at the anode
d. patient skin dose
e. the cooling period required between exposures

Q.1.4 **Centre-tapped transformers are used in x-ray generator circuits instead of simple transformers with two tappings, because**

a. the transformer gives a higher voltage
b. it is safer to wire the mA meter to the centre of the transformer
c. the maximum voltage relative to ground in the high voltage circuit is reduced by 50%
d. mains voltage fluctuations have less effect
e. the electrical power required is reduced by 50%

For answers see over

Answers

A.1.1 a. T—Characteristic photons are not produced below approximately 70 kVp.
b. F—Continuous radiation is produced at all times.
c. F—The shape of the spectrum is independent of mA.
d. F—An ionisation chamber response is independent of energy to a large extent and therefore unsuitable to determine the energy spectrum directly.
e. F—Any spectral hardening due to air is negligible.

A.1.2 a. T
b. F—The area of target that is hit by the electrons does not depend upon filament–anode distance.
c. F—Provided the angle does not change.
d. F—The number of electrons will not alter the area bombarded at the target.
e. F—The area bombarded at any point in time does not change.

Answers b, d and e are correct but only to first order approximations; very small dependence, unlikely to affect practical radiology, may be present.

A.1.3 a. F—The effective energy has no dependence on the mA.
b. F—The amount of scatter depends on kVp with a non-linear relationship.
c. T—Definition of heat units.
d. F—Tube output and thus patient dose will depend on kVp^2.
e. T—As this quantity relates to the amount of heat produced during an exposure it is also proportional to the time required between exposures to allow the heat to dissipate.

A.1.4 a. F—The voltage step-up is governed by the number of turns on each winding and the position of the earth (i.e. the centre tapping) will not affect this.
b. F—The kV meter is wired to the centre of the secondary.
c. T—One side of the circuit will be kVp/2 above ground, the other will be kVp/2 below ground.
d. F—The fluctuations will be unchanged.
e. F—The potential difference and current are unchanged, thus the power will be unchanged.

Questions

Q.1.5 **The interactions that take place within the patient during a diagnostic x-ray examination**

a. are mainly photoelectric interactions
b. are most frequently scattering events
c. always produce an absorbed radiation dose
d. are interactions that take place with electrons in the patient
e. depend upon the kV used

Q.1.6 **The half-value thickness**

a. is the thickness of material required to reduce the intensity of the radiation beam to half its initial value
b. is usually measured in millimetres of aluminium for a diagnostic x-ray beam
c. has a value of approximately 5 mm at 70 kVp for a diagnostic x-ray spectrum
d. can be related to the linear attenuation coefficient of the material used in the measurement
e. is a measure of the quality of the radiation beam

Q.1.7 **Regarding ionisation chambers:**

a. The amount of charge liberated depends upon the chamber volume and the amount of radiation
b. The chamber walls are usually made of aluminium
c. The "free air" chamber is used only as a National standard of exposure
d. The applied chamber voltage is never large enough to produce saturation within the chamber
e. The wall of the chamber and not the gas contributes the major portion of the ionisation that is detected

Q.1.8 **Absorbed dose**

a. is a measure of the energy absorbed per unit thickness of tissue
b. may be measured as watts per kilogram
c. is normally stated in grays
d. may be determined from an ionisation chamber measurement
e. for a given exposure will depend upon the type of tissue

For answers see over

Answers

A.1.5   a. F—The most common interaction in the patient as a whole is the Compton effect.

        b. T—Both coherent and Compton effects are scattering effects.

        c. F—There is no transfer of energy to the patient during a coherent scattering event.

        d. T—Nuclei are only involved at much higher energies than diagnostic x-rays.

        e. T—Low kV will increase the proportion of photoelectric interactions; the likelihood of Compton interactions taking place is almost independent of energy in the diagnostic range.

A.1.6   a. T
        b. T
        c. T
        d. T
        e. T

A.1.7   a. T
        b. F
        c. T
        d. F
        e. T

A.1.8   a. F—Absorbed dose is the energy absorbed per unit mass.

        b. F—It is measured in J/kg.

        c. T—1 gray is equal to an absorbed energy of 1 J/kg.

        d. T—After appropriate corrections, the ionisation in air can be related to the absorbed energy in a given tissue.

        e. T—The absorbed dose will depend upon the mass absorption coefficient of the tissue irradiated.

Q.1.9   Scattered radiation

   a. can have greater energy than the primary beam
   b. will not be detected under conditions of good geometry
   c. is more likely to be present at the detector if the kV is increased
   d. would be very effectively removed by a grid with a grid ratio of 0.1
   e. is removed more effectively by a moving grid compared with a stationary grid of the same construction

Q.1.10   Changing the focus–film distance from 60 to 120 cm has the following effect on the x-ray examination:

   a. The kVp must be increased by approximately 10 kV if the mAs is kept the same
   b. The mAs must be increased by a factor of 4 if the kV is kept the same
   c. The image is magnified by a factor of 4
   d. The geometric unsharpness is reduced
   e. The x-ray field must be increased by a factor of 2 in each direction

Q.1.11   Geometric unsharpness

   a. is minimised by having a small focal spot size
   b. is usually larger than parallax unsharpness
   c. depends on the kV used for the examination
   d. is 0.6 mm if the focus–film distance is 100 cm, the focal spot size is 0.6 mm and the object distance is 10 cm
   e. will be reduced by a moving grid

Q.1.12   The radiation dose to the liver of a patient undergoing a radionuclide investigation is increased by

   a. rapid clearance from the liver
   b. the emission of particles as well as photons by the isotope
   c. long investigation times
   d. poor collimator efficiency
   e. long physical half-life of the isotope

For answers see over

Answers

A.1.9 a. F—Scattered radiation is always of reduced energy.
  b. T—This is the definition of good geometry, i.e. no scatter detected.
  c. T—Although less scatter is produced as kV increases, it has a better chance of reaching the detector.
  d. F—A high grid ratio is required.
  e. F—There is no difference in scatter rejection; movement just removes images of grid lines.

A.1.10 a. F—The inverse square law indicates that tube output must be increased by a factor of 4; a 10 kV increase would not achieve this unless originally the kV was 10 kVp!
  b. T—See answer a.
  c. F—Magnification is reduced as focus–film distance is increased.
  d. T
  e. F—Field size must be reduced but the exact reduction factor depends on the object–film distance.

A.1.11 a. T
  b. T
  c. F—It depends only on focal spot size, focus–film distance and object–film distance.
  d. T
  e. F—See answer c.

A.1.12 a. F—Little dose will be deposited in the liver if there is rapid clearance from the organ.
  b. T—Beta particles (or alphas) travel very short distances and will deposit their energy locally.
  c. F—Once administered, the isotope will deposit its energy independently of the investigation.
  d. T—In order to obtain adequate counts in a given time the activity will have to be increased and thus the dose will be increased.
  e. T—Provided the same activity is administered, an isotope with a long half-life will contain more atoms and the total capacity to create dose will be increased.

Q.1.13 **The following statements are true in relation to technetium-99ᵐ:**

a. The half-value thickness in lead for the 140 keV gamma-rays is approximately 0.3 mm

b. The whole body dose equivalent received by the patient undergoing a bone scan using technetium-99m-labelled phosphonate is approximately 50 mSv

c. The physical half-life of technetium-99 is 6 hours

d. The optimum crystal thickness for NaI detectors in a gamma camera is 0.635 cm

e. The major disadvantage of technetium-99m is that it has low energy particle emissions

Q.1.14 **The CT image**

a. is made up of voxels

b. is made up of pixels

c. resolution is equal to pixel size

d. will have less artifacts due to partial volume effects when the slice thickness is reduced

e. partial volume effect can be reduced if the mA is increased

Q.1.15 **A modern CT scanner**

a. uses several x-ray tubes to acquire transmission data from different directions around the patient

b. uses detectors with at least 60% efficiency

c. produces images with a resolution of approximately 5 line pairs/mm

d. produces images with a minimum detectable contrast of less than 1%

e. can complete a scan in less than 0.1 s

Q.1.16 **Amplifiers of ultrasound signals use swept gain in order to**

a. allow for the different velocity of propagation in the various tissues through which the beam passes

b. compensate for the loss of signal from deep structures due to absorption

c. eliminate signals due to multiple reflections

d. overcome the change in frequency due to moving structures

e. improve axial resolution at greater depth

For answers see over

Answers

A.1.13 a. T—The linear attenuation coefficient of lead at 140 keV is approximately 2.3 mm^{-1}.
      b. F—The dose equivalent is less than 10 mSv.
      c. F—Technetium-99 is stable (compare with technetium-99m).
      d. T—This thickness is large enough to ensure most 140 keV photons are stopped and small enough to preserve resolution.
      e. F—140 keV photons are the only significant emissions; a small number of characteristic x-rays and electrons are emitted but these do not present a problem.

A.1.14 a. T—The display is information obtained from the volume elements or voxels.
      b. T—The picture elements of the display are called pixels.
      c. F—As an approximation, resolution = 1.5 pixels.
      d. T—Narrow slices mean that the probability that a voxel contains only one tissue type is increased and thus there are less partial volume effects.
      e. F—Partial volume effect does not depend upon mA.

A.1.15 a. F—Only one x-ray tube is used.
      b. T—Detectors have efficiencies between 60% and 95%.
      c. F—The best resolution is about 5 line pairs/cm.
      d. T—Contrast detectabilities between 0.3% and 0.5% are obtainable.
      e. F—The fastest CT systems are currently 1 s scan times.

A.1.16 a. F—See answer b.
      b. T—Signal attenuation is path length dependent and therefore the gain is compensated appropriately.
      c. F—Swept gain will not eliminate such signals.
      d. F—Swept gain has no effect on this.
      e. T—Resolution improves because signals that would have been lost are detected.

Questions

Q.1.17 In muscle tissue the velocity of propagation of ultrasound

a. is approximately that in air
b. is directly proportional to frequency
c. is approximately 1585 m/s
d. is appreciably higher than in bone
e. determines the refraction of the beam when the acoustic impedance changes

Q.1.18 The frequency of precession of a magnetic moment arising from nuclear spin is

a. directly proportional to the strength of the external magnetic field
b. known as the Nyquist frequency
c. the same for all materials
d. independent of the temperature and pressure
e. approximately 20 cycles/s

Q.1.19 Regarding MR relaxation times:

a. Spin-lattice relaxation time is usually greater than spin–spin relaxation time
b. In solids T1 is always much larger than T2
c. A relaxation time is a measure of the exponential decay of the magnetic moment
d. A relaxation time is the duration between successive radio-frequency pulses in a magnetic resonance imager
e. Superconducting magnets lead to shorter relaxation times than those measured with resistive core magnets at a given field strength

For answers see over

Answers

A.1.17 a. F—Velocity in muscle is 1585 m/s; velocity in air is 330 m/s.
  b. F—Velocity is independent of frequency.
  c. T
  d. F—Velocity in bone is 2000–3000 m/s.
  e. T—This is the reason for refraction.

A.1.18 a. T
  b. F
  c. F—The frequency depends upon the magnetic field and the gyromagnetic moment which depends upon the material.
  d. T—Depends only upon magnetic field and material.
  e. F—Radiofrequencies are used in the range of kHz–MHz.

A.1.19 a. T
  b. T
  c. F—Magnetic moments return to equilibrium after disturbance by an exponential relaxation process which has a characteristic time period, the relaxation time.
  d. F—Duration between successive signals is governed by the repetition rate and is not the relaxation time.
  e. F—Relaxation times are physical constants at a given field strength.

Q.1.20 Regarding MR:

   a. Spatial resolution in MRI depends on which relaxation time is imaged
   b. MR signals are very weak because there is only a small excess of spin up over spin down nuclei
   c. MR spectroscopy can be used to identify chemical components of a voxel
   d. Each voxel in an MR image contains only one free induction decay
   e. Each nuclear spin gives rise to a free induction decay when disturbed from equilibrium

Q.1.21 These radiographic examinations commonly use cephalad x-ray tube angulation:

   a. AP sacrum
   b. Townes (30 degree FO) view of skull
   c. AP acromioclavicular joints
   d. Apical view of chest
   e. Coned renal areas during intravenous urography in a child following a fizzy drink

Q.1.22 In pelvimetry

   a. in the lateral view a perforated metal ruler is placed at the level of the table
   b. a kVp of between 70 and 80 should be used
   c. an inlet view is useful to show the shape of the pelvis
   d. the position of the placenta will be shown accurately
   e. a 2–3 mm aluminium filter should be used

Q.1.23 In mammography

   a. when magnification mammography is used, the radiation dose to the breast is increased 8-fold
   b. the nipple should always be in profile for standard views
   c. for the axillary view the tube and cassette need to be angled 45°–60° in a craniad direction
   d. dedicated film processing increases the sensitivity of mammography
   e. grids are of particular advantage in imaging the more dense, large breast

For answers see over

Answers

A.1.20 a. F—It depends on the localisation of the signal rather than the type of signal.
      b. T—The excess is only 1.4 parts per 10^6.
      c. T—Some sophisticated MR systems allow spectroscopy to be carried out on selected voxels.
      d. F—Each nucleus gives rise to a free induction decay signal.
      e. T

A.1.21 a. T
      b. F
      c. F
      d. T
      e. F

A.1.22 a. F—It is placed at the level of the natal cleft, parallel to the cassette.
      b. F—90–120 kVp is used.
      c. T
      d. F
      e. T

A.1.23 a. F—The radiation dose is 1.5–4 times that of conventional mammography.
      b. T
      c. T
      d. T
      e. T

Sickles EA (1979) Microfocal spot magnification mammography using xeroradiographic and screen-film recording systems. Radiology 131:599–607

Q.1.24 The former is appropriate to demonstrate the latter:

a. Semi-axial projection of the skull and the jugular foramen
b. 5 mm thick axial CT sections and the internal auditory canals
c. Submentovertical projection of the skull and the foramen rotundum
d. 1.5 mm thick coronal CT sections and the descending portion of the facial canal
e. Magnetic resonance imaging and metallic intraocular foreign body

Q.1.25 On a normal erect chest radiograph

a. the inferior pulmonary veins typically run a more vertical course than the lower lobe pulmonary arteries
b. companion shadows are visible below the clavicles
c. the azygos vein may be up to 2.5 cm in diameter
d. some or all of the horizontal (minor) fissure is seen in about 50%–60% of individuals
e. the carinal angle in an adult is about 100°

Q.1.26 Relating to the heart and great vessels:

a. The right coronary artery arises from the right posterior aortic sinus
b. The non-coronary sinus is the most caudal
c. The right coronary artery is dominant in over three-quarters of the population
d. Septal branches arise from the left anterior descending artery
e. The ventricular septum is best visualised in the AP projection on cardiac angiography

For answers see over

Answers

A.1.24 a. F
          b. F—1.5–2 mm thick sections.
          c. F
          d. T
          e. F

A.1.25 a. F
          b. F
          c. F—Usually up to 0.7 cm.
          d. T
          e. F

A.1.26 a. F—It arises from the anterior sinus.
          b. T
          c. T
          d. T
          e. F—LAO projection.

Q.1.27 **In ultrasound of the normal abdomen**

a. the pancreas becomes more echogenic over the age of 60 years
b. the abdominal aorta is usually seen throughout and has a diameter of less than 2.5 cm
c. the bright white echoes in the renal pelvis and medulla are due to the calyces and uroepithelium alone
d. the diaphragm has a thickness of 3 mm or less
e. biliary sludge may be seen in the gall bladder in fasting patients

Q.1.28 **The gall bladder**

a. normally contains 100 ml of bile
b. fundus becomes continuous with the cystic duct
c. is supplied by the cystic artery
d. is related inferiorly to the transverse colon
e. demonstrates Hartmann's pouch as a normal feature

Q.1.29 **The femoral artery**

a. enters the thigh at the femoral point which is midway between the anterior inferior iliac spine and the symphysis pubis
b. should ideally be transfixed by needle puncture prior to catheterisation using the Seldinger technique
c. may often be more easily catheterised if the catheter is rotated in a clockwise direction over the guidewire
d. should be manually compressed for about five minutes following removal of an angiographic catheter
e. by convention becomes the popliteal artery when it has pierced the adductor magnus

Q.1.30 **Regarding nutrient foraminae and arteries:**

a. That of the radius runs towards the elbow
b. Those of the femur run towards the hip
c. In a minority of individuals, those of the scaphoid are restricted to the distal half of the bone
d. Those of the ilium are Y-shape
e. Those of the vertebrae are confined to the posterior elements

For answers see over

Answers

A.1.27 a. T
        b. T
        c. F—Parapelvic and paracalyceal fat.
        d. T
        e. T

A.1.28 a. F—About 30 ml.
        b. F
        c. T
        d. T
        e. F—*Gray's Anatomy* regards the presence of the pouch to be associated with pathological conditions.

A.1.29 a. F
        b. F—It may be necessary but is not "ideal".
        c. T
        d. F—At least 10 minutes.
        e. T

A.1.30 a. T
        b. T
        c. T
        d. T
        e. F

Q.1.31 The following are true statements:

a. The left renal vein crosses over the superior mesenteric artery
b. The right renal artery crosses anterior to the inferior vena cava
c. The left kidney is related to the jejunum which lies anteriorly
d. The right kidney is related to the duodenum which lies anteriorly
e. The renal artery divides at its first division into superior and inferior branches

Q.1.32 The thyroid cartilage

a. is composed of yellow elastic cartilage
b. lies at the level of the second cervical vertebra
c. has fibrous joints articulating with the arytenoid and cricoid cartilages
d. is the medial wall of the piriform fossa
e. gives attachment to the epiglottis

Q.1.33 The infratemporal fossa

a. contains the mandibular nerve
b. is limited medially by the pharynx
c. communicates with the pterygopalatine fossa via the sphenopalatine foramen
d. contains the maxillary artery
e. communicates with the orbit via the inferior orbital fissure which is between the greater and lesser wings of the sphenoid

Q.1.34 In a PA radiograph of the skull with a 20 degree caudal tilt the following structures may be seen:

a. Foramen rotundum
b. Sphenoidal (superior orbital) fissure
c. Dorsum sellae
d. Crista galli
e. Foramen magnum

For answers see over

Answers

A.1.31 a. F
        b. F
        c. T
        d. T
        e. F

A.1.32 a. F—It is composed of hyaline cartilage.
        b. F
        c. F—Synovial joints.
        d. F
        e. T

A.1.33 a. T
        b. T
        c. F—Via the pterygomaxillary fissure.
        d. T
        e. F—The inferior orbital fissure is between the greater sphenoid wing and maxilla.

A.1.34 a. F
        b. T
        c. F
        d. T
        e. F

Q.1.35 The foramen magnum

    a. is wider posteriorly than anteriorly
    b. transmits the spinal roots of the accessory nerve
    c. on midline sagittal cranial MRI has its anterior limit indicated by the position of the fat pad on the superior surface of the dens
    d. transmits the anterior spinal arteries
    e. transmits the apical ligament of the dens

Q.1.36 These arteries are branches of the internal carotid artery:

    a. Ophthalmic artery
    b. Meningohypophyseal trunk
    c. Posterior choroidal artery
    d. Middle cerebral artery
    e. Middle meningeal artery

Q.1.37 The internal auditory canal

    a. opens medially into the middle cranial fossa
    b. transmits the chorda tympani nerve
    c. is divided into anterior and posterior compartments by the crista transversalis
    d. lies approximately in the coronal plane
    e. is seen on a submentovertical skull radiograph

Q.1.38 Cerebrospinal fluid

    a. is passively secreted by the choroid plexus
    b. flows cephalad from the basal cisterns
    c. is formed at a rate of about 3 litres per day
    d. may flow sufficiently rapidly to create a signal void in the cerebral aqueduct on MR scanning
    e. flows caudally anterior to the spinal cord and cephalad posterior to it

For answers see over

Answers

A.1.35 a. T
       b. T
       c. T
       d. T
       e. T

A.1.36 a. T
       b. T
       c. F
       d. T
       e. F

A.1.37 a. F
       b. F
       c. F—Superior and inferior compartments.
       d. T
       e. T

A.1.38 a. F
       b. T
       c. F—600 ml/day.
       d. T
       e. T

Gado MH, Hodges FJ, Sartar KJ (1987) Hydrocephalus. In: A categorical course in diagnostic radiology – neuroradiology. Radiological Society of North America, Oak Brook, IL, pp 9–20

Q.1.39 **The superior orbital fissure**

   a. lies between the greater and lesser wings of the sphenoid
   b. transmits the ophthalmic artery
   c. transmits the sixth cranial nerve
   d. transmits the maxillary nerve
   e. transmits the inferior division of the third cranial nerve

Q.1.40 **The pituitary gland**

   a. is completely enclosed by dura
   b. possesses a portal circulation
   c. shares the sella turcica with the intercavernous sinuses
   d. is crossed superiorly by the precommunical branches of the anterior cerebral arteries
   e. may be normal if 13 mm in height

Q.1.41 **The following are normal ranges for tissue in Hounsfield units (HU):**

   a. Bone: between 200 and 350 HU
   b. Lung: between -150 and -350 HU
   c. Fat: between -80 and -150 HU
   d. Soft tissues: between 40 and 60 HU
   e. Water: between -40 and -60 HU

Q.1.42 **Regarding imaging of lymph nodes:**

   a. Lower limb lymphangiography routinely demonstrates the internal iliac nodes
   b. Para-aortic lymph nodes 1 cm in diameter are unequivocally enlarged
   c. Reactive hyperplasia and malignant infiltration are reliably distinguished by CT
   d. Intravenous contrast administration produces significant enhancement of normal lymph nodes on CT
   e. Gallium-67 is a useful radionuclide for the demonstration of lymph node masses

For answers see over

Answers

A.1.39 a. T
         b. F
         c. T
         d. F
         e. T

A.1.40 a. F
         b. T
         c. T
         d. T
         e. F—9 mm is the upper limit of normal.

Bonneville JF, Cattin F, Dietemann JL (1986) Computed tomography of the pituitary gland. Springer, Berlin Heidelberg New York.

A.1.41 a. F
         b. F
         c. F
         d. T
         e. F

A.1.42 a. T
         b. F—>1.5 cm on CT.
         c. F
         d. F
         e. T

Q.1.43 Regarding hysterosalpingography:

a. Non-filling of the Fallopian tubes due to spasm may be relieved by intravenous glucagon
b. Intravenous pethidine may be used to relieve pain
c. Salpingitis within the preceding six months precludes examination
d. The technique can be used to show the integrity of a uterine scar following caesarian section
e. The cervical canal should measure less than 10 mm in diameter

Q.1.44 Concerning examination of the neonatal and infant hip:

a. The femoral head is visible at one month on a plain radiograph
b. Screening by clinical examination for congenital dislocation of the hip is accurate in 95% of cases
c. Ultrasound of the neonatal hip clearly displays the femoral head and the cartilaginous acetabulum
d. A 3.5 mHz probe should be used for ultrasound examination
e. Ultrasound has a higher diagnostic yield than plain radiography in examination of the hip

Q.1.45 Regarding micturating cystography in infants:

a. General anaesthesia is usually required
b. About 500 ml contrast medium is usually required
c. Close coning to the bladder area is desirable during screening and taking radiographs
d. Micturition should be observed with the patient standing
e. The use of a balloon catheter is desirable

For answers see over

Answers

A.1.43 a. T
      b. F—Contracts smooth muscle of Fallopian tubes.
      c. T
      d. T
      e. F—6 mm.

A.1.44 a. F—Between 2 and 6 months.
      b. F—50%.
      c. T
      d. F—5 or 7.5 MHz.
      e. T

Leck I (1986) An epidemiological assessment of neonatal screening of dislocation of the hip. J R Coll Physicians Lond 20:56–62

Scott ST (1989) Infant hip ultrasound. Clin Radiol 40:551–553

A.1.45 a. F
      b. F—This is very near to the adult requirement.
      c. F—Otherwise ureteric reflux will be missed.
      d. F
      e. F—Risk of over-distension of the bladder.

Q.1.46 **In the investigation of the source of gastrointestinal bleeding**

    a. a radionuclide study with an injection of technetium-99m pertechnetate may be of value

    b. contrast angiography is useful if the bleeding rate is below 0.5 ml/minute

    c. technetium-99m sulphur colloid is less sensitive than contrast angiography

    d. technetium-99m-labelled red cells are more sensitive in the detection of slow, intermittent bleeding than technetium-99m sulphur colloid

    e. radionuclide studies may have to be repeated several times before showing the site of bleeding

Q.1.47 **Regarding CT of the chest:**

    a. The lung parenchyma may be satisfactorily viewed at a window level of +750 HU and a window width of 1000 HU

    b. The dependent portions of the lungs may normally show increased attenuation compared with the non-dependent portions

    c. The presence of air within the oesophageal lumen is rare in normal individuals

    d. Evaluation of superior mediastinal anatomy is best assessed following intravenous contrast administration via the right arm

    e. Scans are usually obtained in full expiration

Q.1.48 **Ultrasound of the breast**

    a. requires 3.5 MHz transducer

    b. is a sensitive indicator of microcalcification

    c. can accurately distinguish cystic and solid lesions

    d. is of no value in the young dense breast

    e. typically demonstrates acoustic enhancement behind the nipple

For answers see over

Answers

A.1.46 a. T
b. F—above this figure.
c. F
d. T
e. T

A.1.47 a. F—Opinions vary but a level of −750 HU is normal.
b. T—This may mimic or hide pathology.
c. F
d. F—Despite potential artefacts, opacification of the left innominate vein is very valuable.
e. F

A.1.48 a. F—5 or 7.5 MHz is required.
b. F
c. T
d. F
e. F

Questions

Q.1.49 **A satisfactory M-mode echocardiographic examination may not be achieved in patients with**

a. sternal depression
b. emphysema
c. tachycardia
d. pericardial effusion
e. hypertrophic obstructive cardiomyopathy

Q.1.50 **Translumbar aortography**

a. has a higher incidence of complications than transfemoral aortography
b. is usually performed under general anaesthesia
c. is usually performed via the right flank
d. should involve aortic puncture at L2 level
e. is inevitably followed by retroperitoneal bleeding

Q.1.51 **Regarding lower limb venography:**

a. Contrast medium with an iodine content of 420 mg/ml is suitable
b. Tourniquets are applied in order to slow passage of contrast medium through the deep venous system
c. Injection of contrast medium into the long saphenous vein at the groin will opacify the deep venous system
d. The long saphenous vein may be cannulated where it runs posterior to the lateral malleolus
e. Calf massage is recommended to improve opacification of proximal veins in the presence of deep vein thrombosis

Q.1.52 **In dacryocystography**

a. local anaesthetic is unnecessary
b. lipoidol ultrafluid is a suitable contrast medium
c. occipitomental and lateral projections are obtained centring to the superior orbital margin
d. contrast remains in the duct system for about 15–30 s
e. macroradiography is a suitable technique

For answers see over

Answers

A.1.49 a. T
        b. T
        c. T
        d. F
        e. F

A.1.50 a. T
        b. T
        c. F
        d. F—L3 should be used for low puncture and T12 for high puncture.
        e. T

A.1.51 a. F
        b. F
        c. F
        d. F
        e. F

A.1.52 a. F
        b. T
        c. F—Lower orbital margins for both projections.
        d. T
        e. T

Bryan GJ (1979) Diagnostic radiography. Churchill Livingstone, Edinburgh.

Q.1.53   In carotid arteriography by direct cervical puncture

    a. the left carotid artery is usually easier to puncture if the angiographer is righthanded
    b. air embolism is a recognised complication
    c. preliminary views of the cervical artery are unnecessary if an intracranial aneurysm is sought
    d. the posterior wall of the artery should not be punctured
    e. a short bevel needle should be used

Q.1.54   In isotope renography

    a. technetium-99m-labelled hippuran is used for measuring renal plasma flow
    b. diethylenetriamine penta-acetic acid (DTPA) is taken up by the kidneys in exchange for bicarbonate
    c. technetium-99m-dimercaptosuccinic acid (DMSA) is taken up rapidly by the kidneys due to poor plasma protein binding
    d. patients should be dehydrated to improve renal visualisation
    e. fainting is a recognised complication when using technetium-99m-DTPA

Q.1.55   Gastrointestinal haemorrhage can be studied using

    a. technetium-99m-labelled tin colloid
    b. sodium pertechnetate
    c. sodium [^{123}I] periodate
    d. technetium-99m-hydroxymethylpropylene amineoxime (HMPAO)
    e. chromium-57-labelled red cells

Q.1.56   The incidence of significant complications following lower limb lymphangiography with oily contrast medium is increased in patients with

    a. concurrent radiotherapy to the mediastinum
    b. mediastinal lymph node enlargement
    c. significant abnormality of liver function tests
    d. significant abnormality of lung function tests
    e. atrial septal defect

For answers see over

Answers

A.1.53 a. T
  b. T
  c. F—There is a risk of dissection following incorrect needle placement.
  d. F
  e. T

A.1.54 a. F
  b. F
  c. F
  d. F
  e. T

A.1.55 a. T
  b. T
  c. F
  d. F
  e. T

A.1.56 a. T
  b. F
  c. F
  d. T
  e. T—Systemic oil embolism is possible, even with a left to right shunt.

Questions

Q.1.57 Metoclopramide (Maxolon)

a. rarely causes drowsiness as a side-effect
b. is best given orally about 5 minutes prior to barium studies of the small bowel
c. is less likely to produce side-effects in children than in adults
d. is less likely to produce side-effects in patients on treatment with phenothiazines
e. has gastrointestinal effects which are antagonised by anticholinergic drugs

Q.1.58 The following contrast agents are dimers:

a. Meglumine iocarmate
b. Sodium/meglumine ioxaglate
c. Metrizamide
d. Sodium iothalamate
e. Meglumine ioglycamate

Q.1.59 Regarding antibiotics used in radiological practice:

a. Prophylactic nitrofurantoin following instrumentation of the lower urinary tract helps to prevent infection
b. The dose of nitrofurantoin should be increased in patients with severe renal failure
c. Ampicillin may safely be prescribed for patients with established penicillin allergy
d. Gentamicin is contraindicated in patients with jaundice
e. Gentamicin should be given by intramuscular injection

Q.1.60 The following are correct statements:

a. Biliary rather than renal excretion occurs with iodinated contrast media with low protein binding
b. Plasma osmolality is approximately 300 mosmol/kg water
c. Extravasation of low-osmolality contrast media may be painless
d. Gastrografin 50% vol/vol is a suitable oral contrast agent for CT
e. Saline containing gas bubbles is a useful "contrast agent" for real-time echocardiography

For answers see over

Answers

A.1.57 a. T
        b. T
        c. F—Dystonic side-effects are more common in patients under 15 years.
        d. F—Extrapyramidal side-effects again.
        e. T

A.1.58 a. T—Dimer-X.
        b. T—Hexabrix.
        c. F—Amipaque.
        d. F—Conray.
        e. T—Biligram.

A.1.59 a. T
        b. F—It is contraindicated.
        c. F
        d. F
        e. T

A.1.60 a. F
        b. T
        c. T
        d. F—About 3% vol/vol.
        e. T

Examination 2

Questions

Q.2.1 It is sometimes stated that the Compton interaction is one between an x-ray and an unbound electron. This is because

    a. only outer orbital electrons are involved
    b. K and L shell electrons are not involved
    c. only conduction band electrons are involved
    d. the x-ray energy is much greater than the binding energy of the electron
    e. the electron is not within the boundary of the atom

Q.2.2 The range of log exposure within which a satisfactory radiograph is produced is called the film

    a. contrast
    b. characteristic curve
    c. latitude
    d. gamma
    e. speed

Q.2.3 Regarding unsharpness:

    a. Very fast screens have an unsharpness of about 0.3 mm
    b. Fluoroscopic screens can have unsharpness of 0.5 mm or more
    c. Parallax unsharpness is more pronounced when viewing a wet film
    d. For minimum total unsharpness the separate unsharpness values should be equal to each other
    e. Subjective sharpness depends on objective contrast

Q.2.4 When using the "air-gap" technique

    a. obliquely scattered radiation misses the film
    b. an increase in the patient–film distance is required
    c. slow intensifying screens are required
    d. mAs should be increased
    e. an air gap of at least 30 cm is needed

For answers see over

Answers

A.2.1 a. F—See answer d.
   b. F—Any electron can be involved provided d is true.
   c. F—See answer b.
   d. T—Any electron with binding energy much less than the incoming photon energy will appear "unbound".
   e. F—Boundaries as such do not exist but any electron that fulfills condition d can take part in the interaction.

A.2.2 a. F
   b. F
   c. T
   d. F
   e. F

A.2.3 a. T
   b. T
   c. T
   d. T
   e. T

A.2.4 a. T
   b. T
   c. F—Fast screens are required due to increased demands on the x-ray tube and generator.
   d. T
   e. T—Air gaps of less than 30 cm still allow a considerable fraction of scattered radiation to be detected.

Q.2.5 **The dose received by patients during radiography may be reduced by**

a. use of a Potter-Bucky grid
b. use of tube filtration
c. use of high kV
d. use of short focus–film distances
e. use of lower mA

Q.2.6 **Maximum permissible doses of radiation do not apply to patients because**

a. the benefits of x-ray examination should outweigh the radiation risk
b. they are members of the general public
c. their exposure to radiation is only occasional
d. they have a wide range of different examinations
e. they have a wide range of ages

Q.2.7 **Regarding radiation protection from non-ionising radiation:**

a. No biological effects have been observed at ultrasonic intensities of less than 100 mW/cm^2
b. Maximum permissible exposure (MPE) is defined as the level of laser radiation to which, under normal circumstances, persons may be exposed without suffering adverse effects
c. The threshold for effects due to sinusoidally changing magnetic fields in the range 1–100 Hz is above 5 millitesla
d. Whole body exposure to static field strengths of values up to 2000 tesla have shown no harmful effects in human beings
e. The average energy in the ultrasound beam is more damaging than the peak intensity

Q.2.8 **The modulation transfer function (MTF)**

a. of a film screen combination depends upon the focal spot size of the x-ray tube
b. will fall to 0.5 at approximately 4 cycles/cm for CT systems
c. can never take a value greater than one
d. cannot be measured for a gamma camera
e. is a measure of the resolution of an imaging system

For answers see over

Answers

A.2.5 a. F—The use of a secondary radiation grid always increases the dose to the patient.

      b. T—Added filtration reduces the unwanted low energy part of the spectrum thus reducing dose.

      c. T—The attenuation coefficient of all tissues falls with energy thus the dose will be reduced.

      d. F—The number of photons required to form the image and thus the dose is independent of the focus–film distance.

      e. F—The exposure time will be increased to compensate, thus total exposure will be the same.

A.2.6 a. T—This is the assessment made by the person requesting the examination.

      b. F

      c. F—Maximum permissible dose limits apply however the dose is delivered.

      d. F—See answer c.

      e. F—See answer c.

A.2.7 a. T

      b. T

      c. T

      d. F

      e. F

A.2.8 a. F—The MTF of a film screen system is a property of the detector not the source.

      b. T—Most CT systems have an MTF that falls to 0.5 between 3 and 5 cycles/cm.

      c. F—Systems with edge enhancement (xeroradiography and some CT) can give rise to MTF values >1.0.

      d. F—An MTF can be measured for any imaging system.

      e. T—The limiting resolution of many systems occurs at a frequency when the MTF falls to about 0.1.

Q.2.9   Regarding CT quality control:

a. Noise should be estimated by using no more than 10 pixels
b. Image uniformity should be estimated by scanning an air-filled perspex cylinder
c. Slice thickness is measured using an inclined plane made of lead held in the centre of the scanner
d. Low contrast detectability should be an order of magnitude better than the noise on the image
e. The modulation transfer function (MTF) curve will not change with slice thickness

Q.2.10   The following tests should be carried out at the frequency suggested:

a. Film/screen contact should be tested using a test grid whenever the cassette is loaded
b. Sensitometry on the film processor need only be carried out if the type of film is changed
c. Noise and uniformity on a CT image should be tested on a daily basis
d. When a new x-ray tube is fitted one of the tests should be to ensure that the characteristic lines occur at the correct energies in the x-ray spectrum
e. If different length high tension cables are fitted to the x-ray tube, a complete test of the x-ray generator is required

Q.2.11   A modern gamma camera contains

a. a high pressure gas within the photomultiplier tubes to make them more efficient
b. as many photomultiplier tubes as there are pixels in the image
c. a light guide to couple the photomultiplier tubes to the detection medium
d. a caesium iodide (CsI) scintillation crystal approximately 0.64 cm thick
e. a copper filter between the collimator and the scintillation crystal to remove the low energy photons

For answers see over

Answers

A.2.9 a. F—Noise should be estimated from no less than 100 pixels.
       b. F—A water-filled perspex cylinder should be used.
       c. F—An inclined plane made of aluminium is usually used.
       d. F—Detectability can never be better than the noise on the image.
       e. T—The MTF in the image plane is independent of the slice thickness; however it may be difficult to measure when the slice thickness is very small due to the noise on the data.

A.2.10 a. F—An annual test is adequate unless the cassette is damaged or dropped.
       b. F—Sensitometry should be carried out daily.
       c. T—CT systems are prone to daily variations in performance; some systems carry out these tests automatically.
       d. F—Characteristic lines always occur at the same energies.
       e. T—The generator loading will change and thus the generator should be checked completely.

A.2.11 a. F—A vacuum must exist within the photomultiplier tubes.
       b. F—The number of pixels always exceeds the number of photomultiplier tubes.
       c. T—Usually made of perspex and ensures a uniform collection of light from the scintillations.
       d. F—Always sodium iodide (NaI).
       e. F—Except in some research applications electronic energy windows are used to remove unwanted photons.

Q.2.12 The 2-D spatial resolution of a gamma camera

    a. is better than that obtained with a CT system
    b. is worse than the spatial resolution of a positron emission tomography (PET) system
    c. improves when used in the emission computed tomography (ECT) mode
    d. is usually expressed in line pairs per mm
    e. is usually measured from a line spread function by using a phantom of different-sized hot spots

Q.2.13 The noise in a CT image

    a. depends on the scan time
    b. depends on the mA used
    c. will be greater when the slice thickness is increased
    d. will affect the spatial resolution
    e. will make low contrast objects difficult to detect

Q.2.14 In CT scanning the Hounsfield number is

    a. independent of patient size and shape
    b. not related to tissue type
    c. dependent on kVp
    d. not influenced by the mA
    e. independent of the type of detector

Q.2.15 In relation to ultrasound technology

    a. piezoelectric materials distort when subjected to a magnetic field
    b. piezoelectric materials produce a potential difference when distorted
    c. maximum transmission from a transducer occurs when the crystal is backed by air
    d. a crystal with a high Q factor produces an ultrasound pulse with a wide range of amplitudes
    e. the acoustic impedance of a material is the product of the medium density and the wave velocity in that medium

For answers see over

Answers

A.2.12 a. F—The resolution is better with a CT system.
b. T—Spatial resolution of 3–4 mm is possible with PET but gamma cameras usually have values about 6–9 mm.
c. F—There is little difference.
d. F—Spatial resolution is usually expressed as a full width half maximum (FWHM) value of a line spread function in mm.
e. F—It is usually measured using a line source.

A.2.13 a. T—Noise depends on the number of photons detected; anything that increases the number detected reduces the noise.
b. T—See answer a.
c. F—See answer a.
d. F—Spatial resolution is governed by geometrical factors and is not noise limited.
e. T—Low contrast detectability is noise limited.

A.2.14 a. T—Small changes are sometimes observed but the values are related to physical constants.
b. F—Different tissues display different numbers.
c. T—If a CT system is operated at different kVp the attenuation coefficient is different and thus the Hounsfield number will change unless the system is recalibrated.
d. T—mA will not alter the Hounsfield value.
e. T—CT numbers do not depend on the type of detector.

A.2.15 a. F—See answer b.
b. T—This is the definition of a piezoelectric material.
c. T—Due to large impedance difference, energy will be reflected away from the back of the crystal.
d. F—A crystal with a high Q factor produces an ultrasound pulse with a wide range of frequencies.
e. T—This is the definition of impedance.

Q.2.16 **Regarding diagnostic ultrasound, where "soft tissue" excludes gas, cartilage and bone:**

a. The attenuation coefficient of ultrasound in soft tissue when expressed in units of dB/cm is approximately proportional to frequency

b. The attenuation coefficient at a given frequency is the same in all soft tissues

c. The speed of sound in soft tissue is 1540 m/s to within 5%

d. The fraction of intensity reflected by a plain wave of ultrasound at normal incidence at a soft tissue interface is usually less than 5%

e. A decrease in intensity by a factor of 1000 is equivalent to a change of −30dB

Q.2.17 **Regarding simple Doppler ultrasound:**

a. The echoes that are detected in the continuous wave Doppler mode originate from the cellular elements of the blood

b. The Doppler shift frequency increases as the angle between the ultrasonic beam and the vessel at which it is directed becomes less

c. Doppler ultrasound techniques use frequencies in the 15–20 MHz range

d. It is not possible to tell the direction of flow from a Doppler measurement

e. Doppler ultrasound is the only technique able to demonstrate flow

Q.2.18 **The magnetic field in a magnetic resonance (MR) imager**

a. usually has a value of less than 0.1 tesla if the system uses a superconducting magnet

b. is made up of a main magnetic field supplemented by field gradients

c. must be uniform to at least 1 part in 10^6 in order to obtain good images

d. is varied according to the tissue to be imaged

e. is different for taking T1 and T2-weighted images

For answers see over

Answers

A.2.16 a. T—It is approximately 0.9 dB/cm per MHz.
           b. F—Variations greater than 10% are present.
           c. T
           d. T—Impedance values are very similar.
           e. T

A.2.17 a. T
           b. T
           c. F—The usual range is between 2 and 10 MHz.
           d. T—Flow towards gives the same response as flow away.
           e. F—Magnetic resonance can also be used to demonstrate flow.

A.2.18 a. F—The magnetic field usually has a value greater than 0.5 tesla.
           b. T—Gradient fields are used to localise the volume of tissue to be imaged.
           c. T—High quality images will only be obtained in very uniform fields.
           d. F—The field is kept constant during an image.
           e. F—See answer d.

Q.2.19 Regarding magnetic resonance (MR) images:

a. The spatial resolution in MRI is not as high as that obtained with an image intensifier
b. MR images can demonstrate function as well as anatomy
c. MR images do not suffer from the partial volume effect
d. Tissues can be identified in an MR image as relaxation times remain constant for all field strengths
e. MR images are formed by a reconstruction process that is similar to CT

Q.2.20 Quality control of MRI

a. need not be carried out very frequently because there are no moving parts
b. uses the same test tools as those used in CT
c. should include a direct measurement of the magnetic field uniformity
d. must include some measure of the energy imparted to the patient
e. should be carried out at different field strengths with a superconducting system

Q.2.21 For the following radiographic examinations the patient is preferentially in the erect position:

a. AP view of acromioclavicular joints
b. Occipitomental view of paranasal sinuses
c. "Skyline" view of the patella
d. AP view of the pelvis for pelvimetry
e. Laryngeal tomography

Q.2.22 Regarding AP renal tomography in adults:

a. The kidneys are usually visible on tomograms taken 8–11 cm from the table top
b. The more "posterior" tomograms show the lower poles best
c. The kidneys are usually visible on tomograms on which the vertebral spinous processes are clearly seen
d. Tomograms at 14–18 cm may be required to show a transplant kidney
e. Tomograms are taken during gentle respiration

For answers see over

Answers

A.2.19 a. T—Compare with image intensifier resolution of about 3–5 line pairs/mm.
b. T—Flow can be imaged by studying changes in relaxation time.
c. F—All imaging devices that use signals from volume elements to form 2-D images suffer from partial volume effects.
d. F—Relaxation times do not remain unchanged.
e. T—Most systems use a process of reconstruction from projections.

A.2.20 a. F—Quality control should be carried out at regular intervals with frequencies similar to other imaging systems.
b. F—Test tool materials behave differently when used in CT and MR imagers.
c. F—Direct measurements are usually beyond the scope of most clinical departments.
d. F—The energy imparted is so small that it is believed to have no significance.
e. F—Field strength is usually not variable.

A.2.21 a. T
b. T
c. F
d. F—It is the antepartum lateral view which is taken erect in order to estimate the degree of descent of the foetal head.
e. F

A.2.22 a. T—Although there is some individual variation.
b. F
c. F
d. T—There is some variation.
e. F

Questions

Q.2.23 The odontoid peg can be optimally imaged by

a. instructing the patient to open his mouth and phonate "Ah" during the exposure of an AP projection
b. linear tomography
c. autotomography
d. sagittal and coronal reformats of 5 mm thick CT slices
e. T1-weighted sagittal magnetic resonance imaging

Q.2.24 Regarding compression in mammography:

a. Curved or round compression devices should be used to show the posterior portion of the breast
b. Vigorous compression should always be used
c. Compression has no effect on radiation dose
d. Compression decreases geometric blurring
e. Compression allows the creation of a uniform thickness to the breast

Q.2.25 The aortopulmonary window

a. is sited beneath the aortic arch above the left pulmonary artery
b. contains fat
c. is crossed by the recurrent laryngeal nerve
d. contains the ligamentum arteriosum
e. is continuous with the pretracheal space

Q.2.26 The thymus

a. is mainly composed of fat in children and young adults
b. in the neonate, may normally show an undulating lateral margin on radiographs
c. reaches its largest absolute size in the third decade of life
d. commonly shows an "arrowhead" configuration on CT in the adult
e. may atrophy in response to chemotherapy, starvation, or other stresses

For answers see over

Answers

A.2.23 a. T
       b. T
       c. T
       d. F—Slice thickness should be 1.5–2 mm.
       e. F—This is not the "optimal" technique for bone imaging in this context.

A.2.24 a. F
       b. T
       c. F
       d. T
       e. T

A.2.25 a. T
       b. T
       c. T
       d. T
       e. T

Armstrong P, Wilson AG, Dee P (1990) Imaging of diseases of the chest. Year Book Medical Publishers, New York.

A.2.26 a. F
       b. T
       c. F—The largest absolute size is reached in the second decade.
       d. T
       e. T

Williams MP (1989) Problems in radiology: CT assessment of the thymus. Clin Radiol 40:113–114

Q.2.27 The right adrenal gland

a. is separated from the right kidney by the pararenal (Gerota's) fascia
b. at birth, is about one-third of the size of the kidney
c. has a blood supply via a single artery arising from the aorta
d. is normally a posterior relation of the "bare area" of the liver
e. takes up meta-iodobenzylguanidine (MIBG)

Q.2.28 Regarding the liver:

a. A plane extending from the inferior vena cava to the gall bladder fossa separates the right and left lobes
b. Venous drainage from the caudate lobe is via the right hepatic vein
c. The main left portal vein runs directly anteriorly from the bifurcation of the main portal vein
d. The walls of the main hepatic veins are brightly echogenic on ultrasound
e. The ligamentum teres represents the obliterated fetal umbilical artery

Q.2.29 The gastroduodenal artery

a. usually arises from the hepatic artery
b. is closely related to the posterior aspect of the pancreas
c. commonly gives rise to the cystic artery
d. gives rise to the left gastroepiploic artery
e. gives rise to the superior pancreaticoduodenal arteries

Q.2.30 Regarding the hip joint and proximal femur:

a. The lesser trochanter of the femur becomes more prominent with lateral rotation of the hip on an AP radiograph
b. The femoral head epiphysis is entirely within the joint capsule
c. The Von Rosen projection for congenital dislocation of the hip involves the external rotation of the legs
d. The head of the femur in adults is at an angle of about 125° to the shaft
e. Shenton's line follows the inferior border of the femoral neck and the lower border of the superior pubic ramus

For answers see over

Answers

A.2.27 a. F
        b. T
        c. F
        d. T
        e. T

A.2.28 a. T
        b. F—Venous drainage is direct to the inferior vena cava.
        c. T
        d. F—This is in contrast to the portal veins.
        e. F—It represents the obliterated vein.

A.2.29 a. T
        b. F
        c. F
        d. F
        e. T

A.2.30 a. T
        b. T
        c. F—Internal rotation of the legs is involved.
        d. F
        e. T

Q.2.31 **The following accessory ossicles are found in the lower limb:**

a. Os trigonum
b. Os suprapetrosum of Meckel
c. Os epipyramis
d. Fabella
e. Os peroneum

Q.2.32 **In the normal lymphatic system**

a. the normal lymph node may be round
b. the normal lymph node may become enlarged for up to six weeks following lymphangiography
c. para-aortic lymph nodes usually extend beyond the transverse process of the lumbar spine
d. there is usually better filling of the right para-aortic chain than the left on bipedal lymphangiography
e. the cisterna chyli forms from the intestinal and aortic lymphatics

Q.2.33 **Regarding the renal tract:**

a. Six papillae project into each minor calyx
b. A duplex kidney is normally larger than a kidney with a single ureter
c. The ureter of the lower moiety of a duplex kidney is inserted into the bladder superior to the ureter of the upper moiety
d. Renal concentrating ability is maximal at birth
e. Parenchymal indentations of fetal lobulation are situated directly opposite the calyces

Q.2.34 **Regarding the external carotid artery:**

a. The inferior thyroid artery is usually the first branch
b. The internal maxillary artery is a terminal branch
c. The middle meningeal artery is a branch of the internal maxillary artery
d. The main trunk of the proximal external carotid artery normally lies anterior and medial to that of the internal carotid artery
e. Injection of contrast medium into the external carotid artery during angiography is painless

For answers see over

Answers

A.2.31 a. T
      b. F
      c. F
      d. T
      e. T

Keats TE (1984) Atlas of normal roentgen variants, 3rd edn. Year Book Medical Publishers, New York.

A.2.32 a. T
      b. T
      c. F
      d. F
      e. T

A.2.33 a. F
      b. T
      c. T
      d. F
      e. F—They interdigitate.

A.2.34 a. F
      b. T
      c. T
      d. T
      e. F—The conscious patient should be warned of a burning sensation prior to contrast injection – even with non-ionic media.

Q.2.35   The temporomandibular joint

    a. is synovial
    b. has a cavity which is divided into anterior and posterior compartments
    c. is most stable when the mouth is closed
    d. contains a fibrocartilaginous meniscus
    e. is not amenable to positive contrast arthrography

Q.2.36   The submandibular salivary gland

    a. has a main duct about 1 cm long
    b. has a main duct which opens by an orifice at the base of the frenulum of the tongue
    c. lies inferomedial to the body of the mandible
    d. is traversed by the external carotid artery
    e. cannot be visualised using CT

Q.2.37   The following are used in the assessment of cerebral ventricular size:

    a. Evan's ratio
    b. Boogaard's angle
    c. The maximum width of the cellae mediae
    d. The Sylvian triangle
    e. Lysholm's line

Q.2.38   With regard to the petrous bone:

    a. The vestibule lies anterior to the cochlea
    b. The stapes articulates with the short process of the incus
    c. The tympanic membrane is attached to the scutum
    d. The foot plate of the stapes is applied to the round window
    e. The cochlea is a spiral structure normally with $3\frac{1}{4}$ turns

Q.2.39   In a correctly positioned submentovertical skull film, the following are expected to be seen:

    a. The carotid canal
    b. The foramen spinosum
    c. The foramen rotundum
    d. The jugular foramen
    e. The foramen transversarium

For answers see over

Answers

A.2.35   a. T
      b. F—There are superior and inferior compartments.
      c. T
      d. T
      e. F

A.2.36   a. F—The main duct is about 5 cm.
      b. T
      c. T
      d. F
      e. F

A.2.37   a. T
      b. F—This is used to assess platybasia.
      c. T
      d. F—This concerns the disposition of branches of the middle cerebral artery.
      e. F—Lysholm's line identifies the normal position of the cerebral aqueduct on a lateral view of an air ventriculogram.

Burrows EH, Leeds NE (1981) Neuroradiology. Churchill Livingstone, Edinburgh.

A.2.38   a. F
      b. F—It articulates with the "lentiform" nodule of the long process.
      c. T
      d. F—It is applied to the oval window.
      e. F—It normally has $2\frac{3}{4}$ turns.

Swartz JD (1986) Imaging of the temporal bone. A text/atlas. Thieme Medical Publishers, Stuttgart.

A.2.39   a. T
      b. T
      c. F
      d. F
      e. T

Q.2.40 **The cavernous sinus**

    a. contains the abducent nerve embedded in its lateral wall
    b. receives the superior ophthalmic vein
    c. receives the vein of Labbé
    d. contains the trochlear nerve embedded in its lateral wall
    e. receives the superficial middle cerebral vein

Q.2.41 **Regarding CT:**

    a. Hepatic veins are often visualised without intravenous contrast enhancement in normal individuals
    b. Intra-abdominal structures are usually satisfactorily viewed at a window level of +40 HU and a window width of 400 HU
    c. The apparent size of an intrapulmonary mass does not vary with the window level and width used for viewing
    d. The size of the diaphragmatic crura varies between inspiration and expiration
    e. The attenuation value (in HU) of water is identical on different scanners

Q.2.42 **The following statements are correct:**

    a. A 22 gauge spinal needle is longer than a 20 gauge
    b. A 20 gauge spinal needle has a thinner shaft than an 18 gauge needle
    c. 8 French gauge catheters are routinely used for cerebral angiography
    d. A 7 French gauge catheter will normally accept a 0.038 in. diameter guide-wire
    e. 18 gauge needles are routinely used for myelography

Q.2.43 **Regarding CT of the pelvis:**

    a. The insertion of a vaginal tampon is valuable to identify the position of the cervix
    b. The patient should be scanned with an empty bladder
    c. The ischiorectal fossae are poorly visualised
    d. Administration of oral contrast 20 minutes before scanning reliably opacifies small bowel
    e. Identification of enlarged lymph nodes is improved by "dynamic" intravenous contrast enhancement

For answers see over

Answers

A.2.40 a. F—It is related to the internal carotid artery.
b. T
c. F—It drains into the transverse sinus.
d. T
e. T

A.2.41 a. T
b. T—Narrower window widths can be useful for liver lesions.
c. F
d. T
e. F—In practice, the HU "numbers" obtained will be different unless frequent meticulous recalibrations are undertaken.

A.2.42 a. F
b. T
c. F—4, 5, 6 or 7 gauge catheters are used.
d. T
e. F—20 gauge at the most; 22 gauge is perhaps in commonest use.

A.2.43 a. T
b. F
c. F
d. F—A longer time is usually necessary.
e. T—Vascular structures enhance.

Questions

Q.2.44 In preoperative localisation of a breast lesion

    a. syncopal attacks are a known complication

    b. localisation using methylene blue is superior to using a needle and wire system

    c. wires are stable in a fatty breast where they are not anchored to a lesion

    d. two views of the breast should be taken at the end of the procedure to show position of the wire

    e. a space-occupying lesion in the breast parenchyma may be localised using water-soluble contrast

Q.2.45 Regarding estimation of fetal gestational age by ultrasound:

    a. Crown–rump length measurement is more accurate than gestation sac volume estimation in the first trimester

    b. Femur length measurement is considerably less accurate than biparietal diameter measurement in the second trimester

    c. Biparietal diameter measurement is more accurate than an accurate menstrual history in predicting the date of delivery

    d. The most accurate estimation is achieved during the third trimester

    e. Biparietal diameter measurements are most accurate with breech presentations

Q.2.46 In the ultrasonography of early pregnancy

    a. at or before 9 weeks the intracranial contents may appear to be anechoic

    b. the fetal heart beating is normally visible at 3½ weeks menstrual age

    c. the placenta is visible before 8 weeks menstrual age

    d. the coccygeal bud protrudes at 9 weeks menstrual age and may be more prominent than the lower limb buds

    e. the gestational sac at between 4 and 7 weeks menstrual age characteristically has a double outline

For answers see over

Answers

A.2.44 a. T
      b. F
      c. F
      d. T
      e. F

A.2.45 a. T
      b. F—Both measurements are equally accurate.
      c. T
      d. F—Estimation is least accurate in the third trimester.
      e. F—A true biparietal diameter measurement may not be possible in breech presentation.

Chudleigh P, Pearce JM (1986) Obstetric ultrasound. Churchill Livingstone, Edinburgh.

A.2.46 a. T
      b. F—It is normally visible at 4–5 weeks.
      c. F—It is visible before 9–10 weeks.
      d. T
      e. T

Timor–Tritsch IE, Rottem S (1988) Transvaginal sonography. Heinemann Medical, London.

Questions

Q.2.47 Full bowel preparation for barium enema should be avoided when the following conditions are suspected:
a. Hirschsprung's disease
b. Acute exacerbation of ulcerative colitis
c. Cathartic colon
d. Colonic obstruction
e. Irritable bowel syndrome

Q.2.48 For prograde inferior vena cavography
a. anticoagulant therapy is an absolute contraindication
b. bilateral femoral vein punctures are performed
c. asking the patient to perform the Valsalva manoeuvre may facilitate vein puncture
d. the femoral vein cannulation requires that the needle should be directed lateral to the femoral artery pulse in the groin
e. Pertrochanteric intraosseous venography may be carried out in children with bilateral femoral vein occlusions

Q.2.49 In shoulder arthrography
a. low-osmolality water-soluble contrast medium should be used
b. 30–40 ml of water-soluble contrast medium is usually required
c. double contrast examination may be achieved using carbon dioxide
d. the subacromial bursa normally communicates with the glenohumeral joint
e. the needle is inserted with the patient's arm abducted and internally rotated

Q.2.50 Regarding selective renal arteriography:
a. A flush aortogram should be performed before selective catheterisation
b. Systemic hypertension is a contraindication
c. Normal renal arteries constrict following injection of adrenaline
d. Injection of 30 ml of contrast medium containing 300 mg iodine per ml at 10 ml/s is suitable for each kidney
e. Oblique views are rarely of value

For answers see over

Answers

A.2.47 a. T—Colonic distension by faeces facilitates identification of the narrowed aganglionic segment.
  b. T—An "instant" enema may be performed to gauge the extent of the disease.
  c. F
  d. T
  e. F

A.2.48 a. F
  b. T
  c. T
  d. F—It should be directed medial to the femoral artery pulse.
  e. F—There is a danger of growth impairment prior to epiphyseal fusion.

A.2.49 a. F
  b. F—About 6–8 ml is usually required.
  c. T
  d. F—Communication implies a rotator cuff tear.
  e. F—The patient's arm should be adducted and externally rotated.

A.2.50 a. T—It is performed to identify multiple renal arteries.
  b. F—It is a common indication.
  c. T
  d. F—Usually 10 ml at 6–10 ml/s is used. High doses are only justified in patients with renal carcinoma to identify the renal vein.
  e. F—They may help to demonstrate lesions of both extra- and intrarenal vessels.

Q.2.51 **For T-tube cholangiography**

a. *ioglycamide* (biligram) is often used
b. intravenous gentamicin should be administered one hour before
c. a tilting x-ray table is unnecessary
d. rotation of the patient from the supine position may improve visualisation of the common duct
e. autotomography has a recognised role

Q.2.52 **With respect to Duplex carotid sonography**

a. "Duplex" refers to the combination of "B" mode ultrasound scanning and Doppler ultrasound
b. the external carotid artery flow normally arrests or even reverses in diastole
c. an uninterrupted image of the cervical vertebral arteries is readily obtainable using modern colour Doppler scanners
d. blood flow continues in diastole through the normal internal carotid artery
e. the use of colour flow mapping often facilitates the acquisition of a representative Doppler arterial trace

Q.2.53 **In imaging of the lumbar spine**

a. flexing the hips and knees facilitates the acquisition of axial CT sections through the lumbosacral disc
b. a CT scan through the lower lumbar spine 24 hours after an intrathecal injection of Iohexol may prove valuable
c. contrast medium introduced into the lumbar subdural space at myelography is characterised by a failure to reach the cervical levels if the patient is tilted head-down
d. the fourth lumbar nerve root exits the spinal canal cranial to the intervertebral disc between fourth and fifth lumbar vertebrae
e. magnetic resonance images in the midline sagittal plane can image the individual nerve roots

For answers see over

Answers

A.2.51 a. F
b. F
c. F
d. T
e. F

A.2.52 a. T
b. T—This is because the external carotid supplies a "resistive" circulation.
c. F—Bone shadowing interrupts the vascular image.
d. T—This is because the internal carotid supplies a "capacitance" circulation.
e. T

A.2.53 a. T
b. F
c. F
d. T
e. F—A parasagittal image will accomplish this.

Q.2.54 Regarding CT on the lumbar spine:

   a. An axial CT section at the level of the L4/5 disc will demonstrate the superior articular process of L5 anterior and lateral to the lamina of L4

   b. The ligamentum flavum is anterior to the thecal sac

   c. The course of basivertebral veins into the vertebral body can be identified

   d. Intravenous contrast administration will permit identification of the anterior spinal artery

   e. Scanning after myelography is best carried out within 60 minutes of the intrathecal injection of contrast medium

Q.2.55 In peroperative cholangiography:

   a. Control film is unnecessary

   b. Films should be taken after 10 ml of contrast have been injected

   c. Screening should be used routinely

   d. Conray 420 is a suitable contrast medium

   e. It is not necessary to fill both hepatic ducts and their main radicles

Q.2.56 In a patient suspected clinically to have osteomyelitis, these radionuclide scans are likely to be of diagnostic value:

   a. Technetium-99m-methylene diphosphonate (MDP)

   b. Technetium-99m-labelled red blood cells

   c. Gallium-67 citrate

   d. Thallium-201

   e. Indium-111-labelled white cells

Q.2.57 The following radionuclides may be used for diagnostic purposes in nuclear medicine:

   a. Indium-113m

   b. Krypton-81m

   c. Technetium-99

   d. Phosphorus-32

   e. Iodine-123

For answers see over

Answers

A.2.54 a. T
        b. F—It is posterolateral to the thecal sac
        c. T
        d. F
        e. F—Layering of contrast will occur: 3–4 h is optimal.

A.2.55 a. F
        b. T
        c. T
        d. F
        e. F

Dooley J, Dick R, Sherlock S (1988) Imaging in hepatobiliary disease. Blackwell Scientific, Oxford.

A.2.56 a. T
        b. F
        c. T
        d. F
        e. T

A.2.57 a. T
        b. T
        c. F
        d. F
        e. T

Q.2.58 A contraindication to

    a. double contrast barium enema is prior rectal biopsy within 48 hours

    b. hysterosalpingography is recent dilatation and curettage

    c. ascending urethrography in the male is a suspected urethral tear

    d. percutaneous renal cyst puncture is a positive Casoni test

    e. the use of glucagon is diabetes mellitus

Q.2.59 These drugs slow down small bowel peristalsis:

    a. Hyoscine *N*-butyl bromide (Buscopan)

    b. Glucagon

    c. Metoclopramide (Maxolon)

    d. Gastrografin

    e. Codeine phosphate

Q.2.60 Lignocaine

    a. in a quantity of up to 50 ml of 1% solution may be injected to produce cutaneous anaesthesia

    b. is relatively contraindicated in patients with conduction defects of the heart

    c. is used intravenously in the treatment of ventricular tachycardia

    d. causes convulsions in overdose

    e. is metabolised by the liver

For answers see over

Answers

A.2.58 a. T
        b. T
        c. F
        d. T—Any clinical suggestion of hydatid disease is a contra-
            indication to needling lesions.
        e. F

A.2.59 a. T
        b. F
        c. F
        d. F
        e. T

A.2.60 a. F—The maximum is 200 mg, i.e. 20 ml of 1% solution.
        b. T
        c. T
        d. T
        e. T

Examination 3

Q.3.1 Tungsten is chosen as a target material for most diagnostic x-ray tubes because

a. it has a high melting point
b. its thermal conductivity is higher than copper
c. it is able to withstand thermal stress better than molybdenum
d. it has a high atomic number
e. its density is low and therefore the anode can be brought up to speed easily

Q.3.2 Tungsten is chosen as the material for the x-ray tube filament because

a. it has a high melting point
b. it has a high density
c. it gives a large thermionic emission at relatively low temperatures
d. it has a high atomic number
e. the electrons from it can be focused easily

Q.3.3 During a diagnostic x-ray examination the two most important interactions are the photoelectric effect and Compton scattering. The following statements are true:

a. The probability of Compton scattering is the same as probability of the photoelectric effect taking place for soft tissue at approximately 25 keV
b. The probability of either interaction taking place depends strongly on atomic number
c. For most diagnostic x-ray examinations the photoelectric effect will predominate in bone tissue
d. The Compton effect will not create an absorbed dose as it is only a scattering interaction
e. At low x-ray energy the Compton attenuation coefficient is approximately equal to the Compton scattering coefficient

Q.3.4 The spatial distribution of x-rays from the target

a. is only affected by the "heel effect" when the tube is old
b. depends on the target material used
c. depends on the target angle
d. is very different for rotating and stationary anode tubes
e. depends strongly on kV below values of 150 kVp

For answers see over

Answers

A.3.1
  a. T
  b. F
  c. F
  d. T
  e. F

A.3.2
  a. T—Melting point is 3380 °C.
  b. F—Irrelevant to choice of filament material
  c. T
  d. F—Irrelevant to choice of filament material.
  e. F—All electrons are the same!

A.3.3
  a. T—Both coefficients are approximately 0.2 cm^{-1}.
  b. F—Only the photoelectric effect depends strongly on the atomic number.
  c. T—The high atomic number of bone ensures this.
  d. F—The recoil electron will cause radiation dose.
  e. T—At low energy the absorption coefficent is very small.

A.3.4
  a. F—The "heel effect" is present in all x-ray tubes but can become more pronounced as the tube ages.
  b. F—Only the efficiency of bremsstrahlung production and the energy of the characteristic lines depend on the target material.
  c. T—The target angle will alter the degree of "heel effect" present.
  d. F—For first order effects there is no difference; however, pin-hole pictures do indicate more off-focus radiation with rotating anodes.
  e. F—Marked changes are only seen if the generating potential is increased to megavoltage values.

Q.3.5 **Alpha, beta and gamma radiation can be distinguished from each other experimentally because**

   a. they have different values of charge
   b. they cause different degrees of ionisation in an ionisation chamber
   c. they have different penetrating powers
   d. they are never produced at the same time in radioactive decay
   e. they each behave differently in a magnetic field

Q.3.6 **Radioactive decay**

   a. always involves the production of beta particles
   b. that leads to the emission of a positron always produces a nucleus of lower atomic number
   c. constants change slightly with temperature and pressure
   d. half life is the time taken for half the atoms in the sample to be emitted
   e. constant is the probability of the decay of an atomic nucleus per unit time

Q.3.7 **A polyenergetic (heterogeneous) radiation beam**

   a. will always be less penetrating than a monoenergetic radiation beam whose energy is equal to the effective energy of the polyenergetic beam
   b. does not have a unique half-value layer
   c. has equal numbers of photons for all energies in the radiation beam
   d. does not obey the exponential law of attenuation of beam intensity
   e. can only be produced by an x-ray tube

Q.3.8 **Increasing the voltage applied to an x-ray tube increases**

   a. the x-ray output in direct proportion to the increase in kVp
   b. the exposure (mAs) required to produce the radiograph
   c. the skin dose delivered to produce a satisfactory radiograph
   d. the scattered radiation at the detector
   e. the transmission by the patient

For answers see over

Answers

A.3.5 a. T—Alpha has twice the charge of a beta particle and gamma has no charge.

b. F—If they reached the ionisation chamber they would produce different degrees of ionisation, however, the ionisation chamber cannot tell the difference as it does not detect single events.

c. T—Alpha will be stopped in a few millimetres of air, beta will be stopped in a few millimetres of tissue and gamma will pass through several centimetres of tissue.

d. F—Any time difference is too small to be measured.

e. T—Different values of charge cause different trajectories in a magnetic field.

A.3.6 a. F—Beta particles are emitted when a nucleus decays by the conversion of a nucleon into a beta particle and some other particle; other decays are possible.

b. T—A proton has been converted into a positron and a neutron and thus the atomic number has been reduced.

c. F—Constants are constants!

d. F—Atoms are not emitted but atoms decay.

e. T—This is the definition of the decay constant.

A.3.7 a. F—They will have equal penetration; this is the definition of effective energy.

b. T—The first half value layer (HVL) is less than the second HVL which is less than the third, etc.

c. F—A polyenergetic beam is a beam of more than one energy but any distribution of energy is possible.

d. T—Beam hardening occurs and the resulting attenuation curve is not exponential.

e. F—Radioisotopes with more than one energy emission exist, i.e. radium.

A.3.8 a. F—Output depends on kVp^2.

b. F—mAs will be reduced as output will have been increased.

c. F—Higher kV means more penetrating radiation thus less skin dose.

d. T—Although less scatter is produced, higher energy means it has a better chance of reaching the detector.

e. T—Higher kV means more penetrating radiation.

Q.3.9 **Regarding x-ray generators:**

a. The rating of an x-ray tube is the maximum tube current which can be used under a given set of conditions
b. The angiographic and cineradiographic ratings are subject to the limits of the single-exposure rating chart
c. Single large exposures that would cause damage to an x-ray tube are prevented by a thermal cut-out in the housing
d. x-ray tubes run from a falling-load generator are more liable to damage due to thermal shock
e. Self-rectified generators are only suitable for low-power x-ray units

Q.3.10 **Regarding thermoluminescence dosimetry (TLD):**

a. The sensitivity of thermoluminescent materials is increased when impurities are present
b. After irradiation of a thermoluminescent material electrons are trapped in the conduction band
c. A thermoluminescent dosimeter is much smaller than an ionisation chamber
d. The accuracy obtained with TLD is better than that from the use of ionisation chambers
e. Thermoluminescence is the same as phosphorescence

Q.3.11 **A Geiger–Muller tube**

a. has an operating voltage of approximately 100 volts
b. has a mica end window if the tube is to be used to detect alpha and beta particles
c. is more sensitive than an ionisation chamber
d. counts individual events
e. is most commonly used in estimating patient doses

Q.3.12 **The degree of transmission through bone tissue**

a. depends on the attenuation coefficient of bone
b. is much greater than that associated with soft tissue at low kV
c. depends on the density of bone tissue
d. is dominated by the photoelectric effect for photons of energy less than 50 keV
e. is independent of the degree of scattering that takes place

For answers see over

Answers

A.3.9   a. F
      b. T
      c. F—Mechanical or electronic interlocks on the mA, kV and timer selectors are used; thermal cut-outs prevent further exposures of any size taking place.
      d. T
      e. T

A.3.10   a. T
      b. F
      c. T
      d. F
      e. F

A.3.11   a. F
      b. T
      c. T
      d. T
      e. F—It is used primarily for monitoring contamination.

A.3.12   a. T—Transmission is exponentially related to the attenuation coefficient.
      b. F—Bone is more attenuating.
      c. T—The attenuation coefficient depends upon density.
      d. T—At 50 keV the number of photoelectric interactions is approximately equal to the number of Compton interactions.
      e. F—Scattering contributes to attenuation and hence affects transmission.

Q.3.13   Regarding contrast:

   a. Film contrast is decreased when scatter is present
   b. Radiographic contrast between two areas of film is independent of the film type used
   c. The thickness of structures alters the radiographic contrast on a film
   d. Subjective contrast depends on the objective sharpness
   e. The difference in optical density measured at two points on a film is called the objective contrast

Q.3.14   Mottle

   a. is observed only when using intensifying screens
   b. is due solely to the random nature of x-ray production
   c. becomes worse if faster screens are used
   d. can be reduced by using a moving grid
   e. is less likely to be observed if exposure time is increased

Q.3.15   The resolution of an x-ray imaging system

   a. is the smallest diameter high contrast object that can be distinguished from a similar object when they are separated by their diameter
   b. is most often limited by the focal spot size of the x-ray tube
   c. is usually measured in lines per unit distance, often mm
   d. is dependent on the type of detector used
   e. is generally improved by reconstructing the image from projections as in computed tomography (CT)

Q.3.16   x-ray intensifying screens

   a. slow down transmitted x-rays so that they have a much greater chance of interacting in the x-ray film
   b. always worsen the spatial resolution of the image
   c. made of calcium tungstate emit radiation over a wide range of wavelengths
   d. are approximately 10 times thicker than the film emulsion
   e. are used because they are insensitive to scattered radiation

For answers see over

Answers

A.3.13 a. F—Film contrast is the average gradient of the characteristic curve (gamma) and this is unaffected by scatter.
  b. F—Radiographic contrast depends upon film contrast.
  c. T
  d. T
  e. T

A.3.14 a. F—Mottle due to the random spatial production of x-rays could be observed with any detector; screen mottle will only be observed with intensifying screens.
  b. F—Screen mottle may also be present.
  c. T
  d. F—The use of a grid will not reduce mottle.
  e. T—Longer exposure times allow the random fluctuations in spatial distribution of x-ray production to be smoothed out.

A.3.15 a. T—This is one definition of resolution.
  b. T
  c. F—Resolution is usually measured in line pairs/mm.
  d. T—The resolution of the system depends on the focal spot, the distances between focal spot–patient–detector and the detector itself.
  e. F—CT has poorer spatial resolution than conventional radiology.

A.3.16 a. F—x-rays either interact or are transmitted, they can never be slowed down.
  b. T—The radiation produced by the screen spreads out before interacting in the emulsion.
  c. T—The spectrum is continuous from 0.2 to 0.6 μm wavelength.
  d. T—The emulsion is approximately 20 μm thick and the screen phosphor layer is between 70 and 280 μm thick.
  e. F—The screen cannot distinguish primary and scattered radiation.

Q.3.17 Regarding the effect of development on film characteristics:

a. Increasing the temperature of development will increase gamma
b. Increasing development time will decrease speed
c. Increasing development time will increase the fog
d. Increasing development time will not alter the film contrast
e. Increasing the temperature of the development will increase the fog

Q.3.18 The characteristic curve of the film provides the following information:

a. Speed
b. Fog and base level
c. Resolution
d. Latitude
e. Half value layer (HVL)

Q.3.19 In a conventional tomography system

a. the thickness of cut depends on the angle of swing
b. the thickness of cut depends upon the speed of traverse during the tomographic motion
c. linear motion can cause linear striations on the film
d. the most complete blurring of structures above and below the chosen plane is achieved by circular motion
e. the reconstruction algorithm used is usually one involving filtered back projection

Q.3.20 The radiation dose to the patient from a CT examination

a. depends on the scan time
b. of 10 adjacent slices is approximately 10 times the dose from a single slice
c. depends on the type of image reconstruction that is used
d. is approximately 10–30 mSv
e. will increase if scan parameters are altered so as to decrease the noise on the image

For answers see over

Answers

A.3.17 a. T—There is little change after a certain point.
b. F
c. T
d. F
e. T

A.3.18 a. T
b. T
c. F—The characteristic curve displays the optical density obtained for a given exposure; resolution is the ability to resolve two adjacent points and is obtained from the image of a line pair test tool.
d. T
e. F

A.3.19 a. T
b. T
c. T
d. F—Hypocycloidal motion produces the most complete blurring.
e. F—Reconstruction algorithms are only used in computed tomography (CT).

A.3.20 a. T—Long scan times lead to higher doses if all other parameters are unchanged.
b. F—Dose is energy per unit mass and thus does not change if the mass irradiated changes. However, there is a slight overlap between slices and thus a multiple slice examination gives approximately 15% more dose than a single slice.
c. F—Data collection and data reconstruction are independent of each other.
d. T—Some low dose techniques can be as low as 2 mSv but routine scans deliver 10–30 mSv.
e. T—Noise is reduced if the number of photons is increased and thus dose increases.

Q.3.21   In skull radiography

a. the submentovertical (axial) view can be obtained with the patient seated
b. a grid is not normally used
c. the central ray for the occipitomental projection should exit at the level of the lower incisors
d. the Stenver's projection is taken with the patient prone
e. the x-ray beam is directed perpendicular to the internal auditory canal in the Stenver's projection

Q.3.22   Orthopantomography

a. involves the use of a curved cassette
b. produces good visualisation of the midline of the mandible
c. is suitable for radiography of the unconscious patient
d. is performed with the patient opening and closing the mouth during the exposure
e. is performed with the x-ray tube stationary, and the patient and film rotating in opposite directions

Q.3.23   The following structures may be visible on normal mammograms:

a. Lymphatic vessels
b. Lymph nodes
c. Lactiferous ducts
d. Areolar glands (of Montgomery)
e. Cooper's ligaments

Q.3.24   In the anatomy of the respiratory tract

a. the left main pulmonary artery divides anterior to the left main bronchus
b. the left lower lobe lymphatics drain to the left paratracheal lymph nodes
c. normal-sized lymph nodes can be seen on CT
d. the pulmonary veins lie posterior to the pulmonary arteries at the hila
e. the bronchial veins commonly empty into the azygos and hemiazygos veins

For answers see over

Answers

A.3.21 a. T
b. F
c. T
d. T
e. F—It is perpendicular to the long axis of the petrous bone and the internal auditory canal is foreshortened. Thus the fronto-occipital projection in which the beam is perpendicular to the internal auditory canal is to be preferred in the plain radiographic demonstration of the internal auditory canal.

A.3.22 a. T
b. F—The mandible is obscured by the cervical spine.
c. F—The patient has to sit still and co-operate.
d. F—Separate open and closed mouth views are useful to examine the temporomandibular joints.
e. F

A.3.23 a. F
b. T
c. T
d. F
e. T

A.3.24 a. F
b. F
c. T
d. F
e. T

Questions

Q.3.25 The following are anterior relations of the oesophagus:

a. The right main bronchus
b. The hemiazygos veins
c. The descending thoracic aorta
d. The left atrium
e. The right posterior intercostal arteries

Q.3.26 Regarding the pancreas:

a. The normal main duct diameter in the head of the gland is up to 3–4 mm
b. The body of the pancreas lies posterior to the lesser sac
c. The uncinate process lies immediately inferior to the left renal vein
d. The neck, body and tail of the gland develop from the embryonic dorsal portion
e. When patent, the accessory duct opens into the duodenum distal to the opening draining the main duct

Q.3.27 The middle colic artery

a. arises as a branch of the superior mesenteric artery
b. runs in the retroperitoneum
c. supplies loops of jejunum
d. is an end artery
e. supplies blood which drains directly into the inferior vena cava

Q.3.28 The calcaneum articulates with the

a. talus
b. cuboid
c. lateral cuneiform bone
d. medial cuneiform bone
e. tarsal navicular bone

For answers see over

Answers

A.3.25 a. F
            b. F
            c. F
            d. T
            e. F

A.3.26 a. T
            b. T
            c. F
            d. T
            e. F—It opens proximally.

A.3.27 a. T
            b. F
            c. F
            d. F
            e. F

A.3.28 a. T
            b. T
            c. F
            d. F
            e. F

Q.3.29 **The following ossification centres are normally visible at birth:**

a. Patella
b. Manubrium
c. Head of humerus
d. Distal femoral epiphysis
e. Calcaneum

Q.3.30 **Concerning the knee:**

a. The medial meniscus is broader posteriorly than anteriorly
b. Popliteus tendon is closely related to the posterolateral margin of the medial meniscus
c. The anterior cruciate ligament is attached to the anterior intercondylar area of the tibia
d. The anterior cruciate ligament runs anterolateral to the posterior cruciate ligament
e. The suprapatellar bursa lies anterior to quadriceps tendon

Q.3.31 **Regarding the testis:**

a. Lymphatic drainage is via the external iliac node group
b. The epididymis is a posterolateral relation
c. The head of the epididymis lies adjacent to the lower pole
d. Uniform low echogenicity is seen on ultrasound
e. It descends in fetal life through the inguinal canal

Q.3.32 **The left ureter**

a. enters the pelvis by crossing posterior to the common or external iliac vessels
b. is an intraperitoneal structure for part of its course
c. is crossed by the left colic vessels
d. is narrowest at its point of entry into the bladder
e. is crossed anteriorly by the ileocolic vessels

For answers see over

Answers

A.3.29 a. F
        b. T
        c. F
        d. T
        e. T

A.3.30 a. T
        b. F—It is closely related to the lateral meniscus.
        c. T
        d. T
        e. F

A.3.31 a. F—It follows the testicular artery.
        b. T
        c. F
        d. F
        e. T

A.3.32 a. F
        b. F
        c. T
        d. T
        e. F

Q.3.33 Concerning the parotid gland:

a. The parotid duct enters the mouth near the second upper molar tooth
b. The parotid duct is deep to the masseter muscle
c. The external carotid artery divides into its terminal branches within the gland
d. The CT attenuation values of the parotid are normally lower than neighbouring muscle
e. The gland is divided into superficial and deep portions in relation to the course of the facial nerve

Q.3.34 Regarding normal teeth:

a. The deciduous dentition consists of 24 teeth
b. The permanent dentition consists of 32 teeth
c. The enamel is slightly more radiopaque than dentine
d. The periodontal membrane is densely radiopaque
e. The first molar is the first of the permanent dentition to erupt

Q.3.35 The parapharyngeal spaces

a. are easy to examine clinically as they lie superficial to the muscles of mastication
b. are filled with air
c. may be asymmetrical due to varying amounts of normal lymphoid tissue
d. are triangular in shape
e. have smooth and clearly defined margins on CT

Q.3.36 Regarding the cervical spine:

a. In flexion, a distance of 10 mm between the anterior surface of the dens and the posterior surface of the anterior arch of the atlas is within normal limits in infants
b. Anterior displacement of the second cervical vertebra on the third is always pathological in childhood
c. The atlas has no foramen transversarium
d. The interspinous distance is maximal between the second and third cervical vertebrae
e. The uncovertebral joints are synovial

For answers see over

Answers

A.3.33 a. T
        b. F
        c. T
        d. T
        e. T

Smith JRG, King WWK, Tang WYM, Metreweli C (1987) Differentiating tumours of the deep and superficial lobes of the parotid gland by computed tomographic sialography. Clin Radiol 38:345–349

A.3.34 a. F—It consists of 20 teeth.
        b. T
        c. T
        d. F
        e. T

A.3.35 a. F
        b. F
        c. T
        d. T
        e. T

A.3.36 a. F—It should be no more than 5 mm.
        b. F
        c. F
        d. T
        e. T

Harris JR (1978) The radiology of acute cervical spine trauma. Williams and Wilkins, Baltimore.

Q.3.37 The following are constituents of the body of the sphenoid bone:

a. The tuberculum sellae
b. The entire clivus
c. The carotid sulci
d. The foramen ovale
e. Planum sphenoidale

Q.3.38 The trigeminal nerve

a. is readily demonstrated by axial positive contrast CT cisternography
b. supplies motor fibres to the muscles of facial expression
c. originates from the mid-brain
d. arises from the posterior surface of the brainstem
e. supplies masseter

Q.3.39 The facial nerve

a. supplies the muscles of mastication
b. courses posteriorly from the lateral end of the internal auditory canal
c. turns posteriorly from the geniculate ganglion towards the middle ear
d. can be adequately examined by CT in the axial plane alone
e. runs in the medial wall of the middle ear above the stapes and under the lateral semicircular canal

Q.3.40 Cerebrospinal fluid

a. has a long T1 relaxation time
b. has a short T2 relaxation time
c. returns a high signal on T1 weighted images
d. returns a high signal on T2 weighted images
e. surrounds the intraorbital portion of the optic nerve

For answers see over

Answers

A.3.37 a. T
        b. F
        c. T
        d. F
        e. T

A.3.38 a. T
        b. F
        c. F
        d. F
        e. T

A.3.39 a. F
        b. F—It courses anteriorly and laterally.
        c. T
        d. F
        e. T

A.3.40 a. T
        b. F
        c. F
        d. T
        e. T

Q.3.41 Regarding magnetic resonance imaging (MRI):

a. The short TI inversion recovery (STIR) sequence minimises signal from fat
b. Tissues with long T2 give high signal on spin echo sequences with a long repetition time (TR) and long time to echo (TE)
c. Standard inversion recovery sequences are T1 weighted
d. Mascara may give rise to artefacts in head scanning
e. Surface coils are used to improve demonstration of deeply located structures

Q.3.42 In the investigation of hypertension

a. an intravenous urogram should be performed routinely
b. real time ultrasound is useful to show renal morphology
c. Doppler flow studies of the renal arteries are useful at excluding a renovascular cause
d. a DTPA renogram with captopril may be of value
e. renal vein renin sampling has a high false negative rate

Q.3.43 Regarding ultrasound of the fetus:

a. The femur length is taken from the metaphysis to the femoral head
b. The femur length is only accurate before 11 weeks of gestation
c. The ratio between the head and the abdominal circumference is useful to assess maturation from 16 weeks to term
d. The fetal head circumference is less dependent on skull shape than biparietal diameter measurement
e. The crown–rump length can vary with the attitude of the fetus

For answers see over

Answers

A.3.41 a. T
      b. T
      c. T
      d. T
      e. F

A.3.42 a. F
      b. T
      c. F
      d. T
      e. T

A.3.43 a. F—It is taken from the greater trochanter to the lower femoral metaphysis.
      b. F—It is accurate before 14 weeks.
      c. T
      d. T
      e. T

Q.3.44 Regarding hysterosalpingography:

a. It is best performed at about the middle of the menstrual cycle if the patient is certain she is not pregnant
b. Lipiodol is the contrast medium of choice
c. Gentle traction on the cervix prevents foreshortening of the uterine cavity
d. Normal Fallopian tubes may measure up to 5 mm diameter in their middle third
e. Prone views may be helpful to confirm free intraperitoneal spillage of contrast medium

Q.3.45 In ultrasound of the neonatal head

a. the chorionic villi are seen as medium amplitude echoes in the lateral ventricles
b. bones of the base of the vault produce useful landmarks
c. with the transducer in the coronal plane the third ventricle is not usually visualised
d. the parahippocampal gyri can usually be clearly identified as paired C-shaped echoes
e. the cerebral arteries may be identified

Q.3.46 Regarding examination for tracheo-oesophageal fistula in infants:

a. It is best performed with the child in the lateral decubitus position
b. A non-ionic water-soluble contrast medium is suitable
c. Warmed contrast medium should be used
d. Contrast medium is instilled into the trachea
e. Video recording of the procedure is useful

For answers see over

Answers

A.3.44 a. T
        b. F
        c. T
        d. F—The diameter is 1–2 mm.
        e. T

A.3.45 a. F—They are seen as high amplitude echoes.
        b. T
        c. T
        d. T
        e. T

A.3.46 a. F
        b. T
        c. T
        d. F
        e. T

Q.3.47 Regarding angiocardiography:

a. A pigtail catheter is suitable for making pressure or oxygen saturation measurements
b. A catheter with a single end-hole is suitable for left ventricular injections
c. Contrast medium with a low iodine concentration is to be preferred for left ventricular angiography
d. Left ventricular ejection fraction is unreliably estimated during ectopic beats
e. Pressure measurements should be taken before right ventricular angiography

Q.3.48 Regarding intraosseous venography:

a. A Lea–Thomas needle (with a serrated cutting edge) is normally used
b. It is readily performed on an outpatient basis
c. Fat embolism is a recognised complication
d. A film taken 10–15 s after injection of contrast medium is usually sufficient
e. The distal lower limb veins may be demonstrated by injection into the calcaneum

Q.3.49 Regarding the portal venous system:

a. Splenic venous pressure is normally up to 35 cm of saline
b. Venous drainage of the body of the pancreas is mainly to the splenic vein
c. Transhepatic portal venography is helpful in evaluation of portal vein thrombosis
d. The superior mesenteric vein lies to the left of the superior mesenteric artery
e. The superior mesenteric vein is not opacified during the venous phase of splenic angiography

For answers see over

Answers

A.3.47 a. F
      b. F
      c. F
      d. T
      e. T

A.3.48 a. T
      b. F—It is usually performed under general anaesthetic.
      c. T
      d. F—The contrast medium usually clears very rapidly.
      e. T

A.3.49 a. F—It is normally up to about 15 cm of saline.
      b. T
      c. F—The technique requires a patent portal vein.
      d. F
      e. T

Q.3.50 Regarding CT of the pancreas:

  a. Oral contrast administration is unnecessary in most cases

  b. Enhancement of the pancreatic parenchyma occurs following intravenous contrast administration

  c. Opacification of the main pancreatic duct occurs following intravenous contrast administration

  d. The attenuation value of the gland is usually considerably higher than that of the liver parenchyma

  e. Fatty infiltration is commonly seen in the elderly

Q.3.51 In myelography

  a. the supine position provides the optimal column of contrast for examination of the thoracic region

  b. the cervical cord is normally widest between the third and fourth cervical vertebrae

  c. short bevel needles should be chosen

  d. tonsillar ectopia is best sought with the patient prone

  e. the optimal level for lumbar puncture is at the level of L3/4 interspace

Q.3.52 Regarding myelography with iohexol:

  a. The presence of blood-stained cerebrospinal fluid is an absolute contraindication to contrast injection

  b. A 90°/90° tilting table is mandatory for cervical myelography carried out following a lumbar injection of contrast medium

  c. Demonstration of the entire spinal canal is not usually possible

  d. Re-screening may be valuable, 60 minutes after an intrathecal injection

  e. Frontal views of the conus region are best obtained with the patient prone

For answers see over

Answers

A.3.50 a. F
b. T
c. F
d. F
e. T

A.3.51 a. T
b. F—It is widest between C5 and C6 vertebrae.
c. T
d. F—The patient should be supine.
e. T

A.3.52 a. F
b. F
c. F
d. F
e. F—They are best obtained with the patient supine.

Q.3.53 **Sampling of venous blood from the petrosal sinuses**

    a. is valuable in the diagnosis of Cushing's syndrome

    b. should be performed simultaneously from both inferior petrosal sinuses

    c. is ideally performed by internal jugular venous puncture(s)

    d. requires the catheter tip to be advanced 1 cm distal to the inferior petrosal sinus orifice

    e. is unnecessary if high definition, intravenous contrast enhanced coronal CT of the pituitary gland utilising 1.5 mm sections is normal

Q.3.54 **It is possible to identify the following vascular structures on routine cranial CT utilising 10 mm thick axial slices after a bolus intravenous injection of 50 ml of iohexol 300:**

    a. The thalamostriate veins

    b. The pericallosal artery

    c. The internal cerebral vein

    d. The anterior choroidal artery

    e. The inferior sagittal sinus

Q.3.55 **Regarding technetium-99m-labelled microspheres:**

    a. After intravenous injection, they lodge mostly in the pulmonary capillaries

    b. Anaphylactic reactions are common with intravenous usage

    c. They provide a useful way of labelling white blood cells

    d. They have been used to study right-to-left cardiopulmonary shunts

    e. They have a more uniform particle size than albumin macroaggregates

Q.3.56 **The following substances can be used to study pulmonary ventilation:**

    a. Xenon-133

    b. Technetium-99m–diethylenetriamine penta-acetic acid (DTPA) aerosols

    c. Nebulised indium-113m ferric hydroxide

    d. Technegas

    e. Iodine-131 vapour

For answers see over

Answers

A.3.53 a. T
       b. T
       c. F—A perfemoral approach is used.
       d. F
       e. F

Doppman JL, Oldfield E, Krudy AG, et al. (1984) Petrosal sinus sampling for Cushing's syndrome. Anatomical and technical considerations. Radiology 150:99–103

A.3.54 a. T
       b. T
       c. T
       d. F
       e. F

A.3.55 a. F
       b. F
       c. F
       d. T
       e. T

A.3.56 a. T
       b. T
       c. F
       d. T
       e. F

Q.3.57 A contraindication to

a. lumbar myelography is papilloedema
b. percutaneous renal puncture is pyonephrosis
c. translumbar aortography is hypertension
d. barium reduction of intussusception is duration of symptoms greater than 6 hours
e. cerebral angiography is raised intracranial pressure

Q.3.58 Venous air embolism

a. is a recognised complication of percutaneous lung biopsy
b. may complicate contrast-enhanced CT
c. is commonly asymptomatic
d. may be associated with an audible cardiac murmur
e. is treated by giving oxygen and turning the patient into the right lateral decubitus position

Q.3.59 Respiratory depression due to the following drugs can be reversed with naloxone (Narcan):

a. Dextropropoxyphene
b. Pentazocine
c. Pethidine
d. Buprenorphine
e. Morphine

Q.3.60 Desirable properties of barium suspensions for double contrast barium meal studies include

a. large particle size
b. high density
c. incorporation of an anti-foaming agent
d. high viscosity
e. stability at acid pH

For answers see over

Answers

A.3.57 a. T—There may be raised intracranial pressure.
      b. F—Percutaneous drainage under antibiotic cover may be life
          saving.
      c. T
      d. F—24 hours is usually quoted.
      e. F

A.3.58 a. T
      b. T
      c. T
      d. T
      e. F—The patient should be in the left lateral decubitus
          position, preferably head down.

Woodring JH, Fried AM (1988) Non-fatal venous air embolism after
contrast-enhanced CT. Radiology 167:405–407

A.3.59 a. T
      b. T
      c. T
      d. T
      e. T

A.3.60 a. F
      b. T
      c. T
      d. F
      e. T

Examination 4

Q.4.1 **Gamma rays are**

    a. always emitted when a nucleus decays
    b. the same as characteristic x-rays
    c. easily stopped in a few centimetres of tissue
    d. indirectly ionising particles
    e. emitted when a nucleus returns to its ground state

Q.4.2 **Isotopes of an element**

    a. have the same atomic number
    b. have the same mass number
    c. are radioactive
    d. have the same number of neutrons
    e. all have the same half-life

Q.4.3 **The energy required to remove an electron from an atom**

    a. is called the rest mass energy
    b. depends on which shell the electron has been ejected from
    c. is called the binding energy
    d. is called the excitation energy
    e. is the energy at which absorption edges occur

Q.4.4 **The quantity of x-ray photons emitted from an x-ray tube**

    a. depends upon the kVp used
    b. will be greater for a tungsten target than for a molybdenum target tube provided all other factors remain unchanged
    c. will be doubled if the mA is halved and the kVp doubled
    d. depends on the degree of filtration
    e. depends on the distance between the anode and cathode

For answers see over

Answers

A.4.1 a. F—Some nuclear decay schemes do not give rise to gamma emission.
   b. F—Gamma rays are due to nuclear transitions; characteristic x-rays are due to electron transitions.
   c. F—Gamma rays obey an exponential law of attenuation.
   d. F—Gamma rays are directly ionising photons.
   e. T—An excited nucleus returning to its unexcited (ground) state will emit gamma rays.

A.4.2 a. T
   b. F
   c. F
   d. F
   e. F

A.4.3 a. F—Rest mass energy is the energy equivalent of an electron at rest.
   b. T
   c. T
   d. F
   e. T

A.4.4 a. T
   b. T
   c. T—Output is directly proportional to mA and proportional to kVp².
   d. T—Filtration always reduces the quantity of photons.
   e. F—The quantity of photons depends on the number of electrons hitting the target. As a vacuum exists between the anode and cathode and the electron beam is focused (no divergence), there should be no change in the number of electrons passing between them as the distance increases.

Q.4.5 **Regarding the dissipation of heat from x-ray tubes:**

a. Heat is transferred by conduction from the focal spot to the body of the anode
b. Heat is transferred by radiation from the focal spot to the glass wall of the tube
c. The oil in the tube housing acts as both an insulator and as a cooling agent
d. Heat is transferred by convection through the oil
e. With a rotating anode very little heat can be dissipated by conduction along the anode stem

Q.4.6 **An x-ray tube is immersed in oil to**

a. filter the beam
b. provide lubrication
c. reduce the shielding required
d. provide electrical insulation
e. protect the tube from mechanical shock

Q.4.7 **The effective energy of the x-ray beam from a constant potential generator is**

a. higher than that from a pulsating potential generator of the same kVp
b. equal to the kVp
c. lower than that from a capacitor discharge generator of the same kVp
d. the same as the energy of the monoenergetic source that has the same penetrating power
e. half the kVp

For answers see over

Answers

A.4.5 a. T
 b. T
 c. T
 d. T
 e. T

A.4.6 a. F
 b. F
 c. F
 d. T
 e. F

Answers a and to a small extent c are consequences of the introduction of oil, but the real reason for its introduction is the electrical insulation it provides.

A.4.7 a. T—Because a greater proportion of the exposure time is spent at the kVp.
 b. F—Effective energy is approximately 1/3 kVp.
 c. F—Capacitor discharge generators have falling kVp during the exposure thus the effective energy will be lower.
 d. T—This is the definition of effective energy.
 e. F—Effective energy is approximately 1/3 kVp.

Q.4.8   In a falling load generator

    a. the operator controls the tube current but the generator selects the maximum kV that does not exceed the tube loading

    b. the patient is exposed to a very short trial exposure from which the optimum exposure is estimated

    c. the kV and mA are automatically adjusted when the load on the National Grid becomes greater

    d. the mA is varied during the exposure

    e. the temperature of the x-ray target is maintained at as high a temperature as possible

Q.4.9   A spinning top test tool

    a. is used to test the exposure timer on any pulsed x-ray generator

    b. must be rotated at a known speed if a constant potential generator is tested

    c. is suitable for testing any length of exposure time

    d. can be used to measure the speed of a film screen combination if it has a synchronous motor

    e. will generate 6 spots per second for a 3-phase fully rectified generator

Q.4.10   In radiation protection

    a. stochastic effects are defined as biological effects whose incidence is some function of the dose received

    b. the effective dose equivalent for irradiation of the body by x-rays is the same as the skin dose

    c. the dose limit for members of the public is 5 mSv in a year

    d. the transmission of 100 keV x-rays through a 0.25 mm Pb-equivalent lead rubber apron is less than 1%

    e. the quality factor is measured in half value layers (HVL) of aluminium

For answers see over

Answers

A.4.8   a. F
      b. F—The patient should never be exposed unless diagnostic information is produced.
      c. F—This correction is carried out by the autotransformer.
      d. T
      e. T

A.4.9   a. T—Only pulsed systems will provide individual dots that can be counted and thus converted into an exposure time.
      b. T—The length of the arc can be used if constant speed is known.
      c. F—Long exposures allow the top to complete more than one rotation thus superimposing the dots.
      d. F—Speed of film screen combination is not related to exposure timer.
      e. F—6 dots will be generated 50 times per second.

A.4.10   a. T
      b. F—Skin dose is the dose received by the skin; dose equivalent weights the absorbed dose to allow for the various factors which might affect the biological effectiveness.
      c. T
      d. F—100 keV transmission is about 20%; 100 kV transmission is about 0.05%.
      e. F—Quality factor has no units.

Q.4.11 The total linear attenuation coefficient

    a. is the same as the mass absorption coefficient
    b. depends on the physical density
    c. is the fractional reduction in energy per unit thickness
    d. is the same for all materials at a given energy
    e. is measured in units of m^2/kg

Q.4.12 A scintillation detector

    a. detects radiation through the conversion of x-ray energy into near-visible photons
    b. produces a pulse whose height is proportional to the energy of the photon detected
    c. is normally operated in the "plateau" region
    d. often has impurities added to the scintillator to improve its performance
    e. is very efficient at detecting x-rays

Q.4.13 The quality factor in diagnostic radiology

    a. is the ratio of kVp to effective energy
    b. is measured in units of half value (HV) thickness
    c. is synonymous with relative biological effectiveness (RBE)
    d. is in the range of 5 to 10
    e. in a CT image is larger than that associated with conventional radiology

Q.4.14 In macroradiography

    a. a tube with a focal spot of less than 0.4 mm is required
    b. a large film–patient distance is used
    c. a high mA generator is required
    d. fast screens can be used because grain size is less important
    e. movement artifacts are increased

For answers see over

Answers

A.4.11 a. F—Attenuation includes the effects of scatter and absorption and the linear coefficient is equal to the (mass coefficient × density).
b. T—The total linear attenuation coefficient is directly proportional to the physical density.
c. F—It is the fractional reduction in intensity per unit thickness.
d. F—It has different values for different tissues.
e. F—It has units of m^{-1}; the mass coefficient has units of m^2/kg.

A.4.12 a. T
b. T
c. F—A clear "plateau" region does not exist with a scintillation detector.
d. T—Most sodium iodide scintillators are thallium activated.
e. T—The attenuation coefficient of most scintillators is high and thus nearly all photons are stopped in the scintillator.

A.4.13 a. F
b. F
c. T
d. F—In the diagnostic x-ray range the quality factor is usually taken as 1.0.
e. F—Quality factor is associated with the radiation beam and not the image quality.

A.4.14 a. T
b. T
c. T—Exposure time needs to be as short as possible thus high mA.
d. T—Image resolution is not limited by grain size.
e. T

Questions

Q.4.15 **The value of the gamma of a processed photographic emulsion**

    a. is a measure of the contribution to contrast that the film makes
    b. is usually between 10 and 30
    c. is expressed in millilamberts
    d. is dependent on the viewing conditions
    e. is dependent on the processing conditions

Q.4.16 **Radiographic contrast is decreased by**

    a. increasing the kV
    b. increasing the focus–patient distance
    c. increasing the patient–film distance
    d. increasing the field size
    e. increasing the added filtration

Q.4.17 **Intensifying screens used in diagnostic x-ray departments**

    a. contain phosphor crystals embedded in emulsion
    b. have more phosphor crystals the faster the screen type
    c. have different types of crystals that depend upon the type of film to be used
    d. contain dyes to prevent cross-over
    e. are thicker than the radiographic emulsion

Q.4.18 **Regarding electrostatic image recording processes:**

    a. The spatial resolution of a xeroradiographic image is better than that recorded on a film/screen combination
    b. The latitude in xeroradiography is very large
    c. Ionography is another word for xeroradiography
    d. Edge-enhancement is usually present in xeroradiographic images
    e. Electrostatic recording methods use electrons rather than x-rays to produce the image

For answers see over

Answers

A.4.15 a. T
b. F—Gamma is usually in the range 0.5–3.0.
c. F—Gamma has no units.
d. F—Gamma is a property of the film and its processing only.
e. T

A.4.16 a. T
b. F—Contrast will not depend on the distance between the source and patient.
c. F—Contrast will be increased due to removal of scatter at the film (air-gap technique).
d. T—Increased scatter will reduce contrast.
e. T—Beam quality will be increased thus less contrast.

A.4.17 a. F—Contains crystals but not in emulsion.
b. T—Packing density and/or thickness of screen will change.
c. T—Rare earth screens contain different crystals.
d. F—Dye is present in the base of radiographic film to prevent cross-over.
e. T—Screens are approximately 10 times thicker than emulsion.

A.4.18 a. T—Film/screen about 5–8 line pairs/mm, xeroradiography about 12–20 line pairs/mm.
b. T—Exposure latitude sufficient to allow soft tissue borders and bony structures to be imaged with same exposure.
c. F—Ionography generally uses a gas as the active element of the detector.
d. T—It arises due to the development process.
e. F—Only the detector is charged.

Q.4.19 Secondary radiation grids

    a. are usually made of lead strips with air between them
    b. increase the dose to the patient
    c. can be placed both sides of the patient to cut down scatter even further
    d. that are focused must be focused on the patient
    e. improve contrast and spatial resolution

Q.4.20 A digital fluoroscopic system

    a. contains an analogue to digital converter
    b. can be used to produce computerised tomography images
    c. contains a digital to analogue converter
    d. produces images with approximately the same spatial resolution as xeroradiographic plates
    e. uses an intensifier with a caesium iodide input screen

Q.4.21 The following are appropriate centering points for radiographic examinations:

    a. AP thumb – scaphoid
    b. Infero-superior clavicle – head of humerus
    c. AP open-mouth atlantoaxial joint – tip of mandible
    d. Dorso-plantar foot – navicular
    e. Lateral oblique temporomandibular joint – contralateral external auditory meatus

Q.4.22 In dental radiography

    a. the occlusal plane is horizontal
    b. the central ray should be perpendicular to a line bisecting the angle between tooth and film
    c. intraoral and occlusal films are non-screen in type
    d. lead markers are used for orientation
    e. it is permissible for the radiographer to hold a dental film in position whilst exposures are made

For answers see over

Answers

A.4.19 a. F—They are usually made of alternate strips of lead and plastic or aluminium.

b. T—Some primary radiation is also removed by a grid and thus the patient exposure must be increased to compensate for this.

c. F—The air between source and patient does not create significant scatter.

d. F—They should be positioned so that they are focused on the focal spot.

e. F—They improve contrast but not spatial resolution.

A.4.20 a. T

b. F—CT images require many projections taken at different orientations; this is not possible with clinical digital fluoroscopy systems.

c. T

d. F—Spatial resolution in digital fluoroscopy is much poorer than that associated with xeroradiography.

e. T

A.4.21 a. F—First metacarpophalangeal joint.

b. F—Middle of clavicle

c. F—Through the mouth.

d. T

e. F—Equivalent to the ipsilateral external auditory meatus.

A.4.22 a. T

b. T

c. T

d. F

e. F

Q.4.23 **The following are demonstrated on left posterior oblique views of the pelvis:**

    a. Right sacroiliac joint
    b. Left pubic rami
    c. Distal right ureter on intravenous urography
    d. Anterior column of the right acetabulum
    e. Left pars interarticularis of the fifth lumbar vertebra

Q.4.24 **Regarding skull radiography and anatomy:**

    a. The anthropological baseline and Reid's baseline are one and the same
    b. Chamberlain's line joins the odontoid tip and the lowermost margin of the occipital squame
    c. The internal auditory canal opens into the middle fossa
    d. Boogaard's angle should be no greater than about 140 degrees
    e. The optic canal opens inferior and medial to the anterior clinoid process

Q.4.25 **Regarding the oesophagus:**

    a. It is crossed by the left main bronchus
    b. The abdominal portion is 1–3 cm long
    c. The ampulla lies below the diaphragm at rest
    d. The abdominal portion lies in a groove on the posterior surface of the liver
    e. Two sling fibres of inner stomach muscle are attached to the oesophagus at the oesophagogastric junction

Q.4.26 **The azygos fissure**

    a. is usually left sided
    b. occurs at the lung apex
    c. consists of four pleural layers
    d. occurs in 5% of the general population
    e. normally contains the hemiazygos vein

For answers see over

Answers

A.4.23 a. T
    b. F
    c. T
    d. T
    e. T

A.4.24 a. T
    b. F—This is describing McGregor's line.
    c. F—It opens into the posterior fossa.
    d. T
    e. T

A.4.25 a. T
    b. T
    c. F
    d. T
    e. T

A.4.26 a. F
    b. T
    c. T
    d. F—It occurs in <1%.
    e. F

Grainger RG, Allison DJ (1986) Diagnostic radiology. Churchill Livingstone, Edinburgh.

Q.4.27 Psoas major muscle

   a. inserts into the greater trochanter of the femur
   b. is a posterior relation of the capsule of the hip joint
   c. is a posterior relation of the ureter
   d. has a lateral margin approximately parallel to the long axis of the ipsilateral kidney
   e. contains the lumbar nerve plexus within its substance posteriorly

Q.4.28 Fat

   a. is of low signal intensity on T1 weighted magnetic resonance images
   b. facilitates identification of the adrenal glands on CT
   c. if excessive, may degrade ultrasound images
   d. is a common cause of abnormal widening of the postrectal space on barium enema
   e. has an attenuation value of about +50 to +100 HU on CT

Q.4.29 In the abdomen

   a. the hepatic veins drain to the inferior vena cava via the "bare area" of the liver
   b. the falciform ligament marks the division between the left and right lobes of the liver
   c. the gastrophepatic ligament forms part of the anterior wall of the lesser sac
   d. the superior aspect of the lesser sac extends to the level of the diaphragmatic crura
   e. the lateroconal fascia fuses with the posterior parietal peritoneum

Q.4.30 Ossification centres of the following bones are often multi-centric:

   a. Tarsal navicular
   b. The cuboid
   c. The capitate
   d. The humeral head
   e. The acromion

For answers see over

Answers

A.4.27 a. F
b. F
c. T
d. T
e. T

A.4.28 a. F—It shares with chronic haemorrhage the property of returning a high signal on both T1 and T2 weighted MR images.
b. T—They may be difficult to identify in children and thin adults.
c. T
d. T
e. F—The attenuation value is variable but usually −100 to −20 HU.

A.4.29 a. T
b. F
c. T
d. T
e. T

A.4.30 a. F
b. F
c. F
d. F
e. T

Q.4.31   Regarding the elbow joint:

a. Three types of movement are possible
b. The radial head articulates with the capitulum
c. In a lateral radiograph a fat-pad is readily seen which is normally closely applied to the anterior surface of the humerus
d. The ulnar nerve is an anterior relation, within the antecubital fossa
e. Arthrography is accomplished by entering the joint between the capitellum and radial head

Q.4.32   Venous drainage of the left kidney

a. is by multiple veins in a small minority of people
b. is a superior relation of the third (transverse) portion of the duodenum
c. when retroaortic, usually runs superiorly and to the right from the renal hilum to the inferior vena cava
d. usually does not receive the venous drainage from the left adrenal gland
e. usually lies anterior to the arterial supply to the kidney

Q.4.33   The urinary bladder

a. is entirely intraperitoneal
b. normally has a maximum capacity of about 1.5 litres
c. at birth, lies in a relatively higher position than in the adult
d. in the male, is an anterior relation of the seminal vesicles
e. contains a triangular portion, the trigone, bounded by the internal urethral orifice and the ureteric orifices

Q.4.34   Regarding the uterus:

a. The attitude is normally anteverted and anteflexed
b. On ultrasound, the uterine cavity shows as a bright central echo
c. On a longitudinal ultrasound scan, the internal os lies in line with the angle between the trigone and the postero-superior wall of the bladder
d. It has no peritoneal covering
e. It is a posterior relation of the rectum

For answers see over

Answers

A.4.31 a. F
        b. T
        c. T
        d. F
        e. T

A.4.32 a. T
        b. T
        c. F—It runs inferiorly and to the right.
        d. F
        e. T

A.4.33 a. F
        b. F—Maximum capacity is normally about 500–700 ml.
        c. T
        d. T
        e. T

A.4.34 a. T
        b. T
        c. T
        d. F
        e. F

Q.4.35 The brachial plexus

a. is usually derived from the anterior primary rami of C5, 6, 7, 8 and T1 nerve roots
b. consists of upper, middle and lower trunks
c. consists of cords named according to their arrangement around the subclavian artery
d. lies in the posterior triangle of the neck
e. has roots which can be reliably identified on intravenous contrast enhanced axial CT using the scalene muscles as landmarks

Q.4.36 These basal skull foraminae transmit cranial nerves:

a. Foramen ovale
b. Foramen lacerum
c. Foramen rotundum
d. Foramen spinosum
e. Anterior condylar canal

Q.4.37 The following are normally branches of the middle cerebral artery:

a. The artery of Heubner
b. The anterior choroidal artery
c. The posterior choroidal artery
d. The pericallosal artery
e. The lenticulostriate arteries

Q.4.38 Regarding the skull in childhood:

a. In the normal neonate overlapping of the cranial bones may occur
b. Vascular impressions in the skull vault are present in the neonate
c. Closure of the posterior fontanelle precedes closure of the anterior fontanelle
d. A metopic suture passes upwards and medially from the lower part of the occipital bone
e. Convolutional markings on the vault in childhood are often more prominent than in the adult skull

For answers see over

Answers

A.4.35 a. T
        b. T
        c. F—They are arranged around the axillary artery.
        d. T
        e. T

Cooke J, Cooke D, Parsons C (1988) The anatomy and pathology of the brachial plexus as demonstrated by computed tomography. Clin Radiol 39:595–601

A.4.36 a. T
        b. F
        c. T
        d. F
        e. T—This is the hypoglossal canal.

A.4.37 a. F—This is a branch of the anterior cerebral artery.
        b. F—A branch of the internal carotid artery.
        c. F—A branch of the posterior cerebral artery.
        d. F—A branch of the anterior cerebral artery.
        e. T

A.4.38 a. T
        b. F
        c. T
        d. F—This is the mendosal suture.
        e. T

Q.4.39 Regarding the third ventricle:

a. The lamina terminalis is part of the anterior wall of the third ventricle
b. The massa intermedia is a white matter tract
c. The chiasmatic or supraoptic recess lies anterior to the infundibular recess
d. The habenular commissure is posterior to the pineal gland
e. The foramina of Magendie connect lateral and third ventricles

Q.4.40 The optic canal

a. is formed entirely by the greater wing of the sphenoid bone
b. transmits the ophthalmic artery which is inferior to the optic nerve within the canal
c. is seen within the lower outer quadrant of the orbit in a correctly positioned optic canal projection ("the four point landing")
d. transmits the superior ophthalmic vein
e. connects the orbital apex with the suprasellar cistern

Q.4.41 On "dynamic" contrast-enhanced CT scanning

a. corticomedullary differentiation in the kidney is possible
b. inhomogeneous enhancement of the spleen may be normal
c. inhomogeneous enhancement of the liver may be normal
d. poor enhancement of the infrarenal inferior vena cava may be normal
e. the bowel wall enhances

Q.4.42 In video cystourography

a. a catheter line is used in the rectum
b. a tiny epidural catheter is inserted alongside the bladder catheter
c. the patient's bladder is filled in the erect position
d. the patient is asked to cough before voiding
e. in normal patients the detrusor only contracts on voluntary voiding

For answers see over

Answers

A.4.39 a. T
        b. F—It is a grey matter tract.
        c. T
        d. F
        e. F—They are connected by the foramina of Monro.

A.4.40 a. F
        b. T
        c. T
        d. F
        e. T

A.4.41 a. T
        b. T
        c. F
        d. T
        e. T

A.4.42 a. T
        b. T
        c. F
        d. T
        e. T

Q.4.43   In Doppler ultrasound of the ovaries

    a. it is easy to detect Doppler signals from an active ovary

    b. an ovary with the dominant follicle develops increased blood flow with continuous diastolic flow

    c. there are high impedance signals with evidence of diastolic flow early in the menstrual cycle before day 10

    d. the presence of active flow to the corpus luteum is seen in pregnancy

    e. after day 23 there is rapid reversion to conditions existing at the beginning of the cycle

Q.4.44   In children

    a. the adrenal cortex involutes rapidly following the neonatal period

    b. an abdominal lymph node measuring 1 cm in diameter on CT is unequivocally normal

    c. the renal outline is more clearly seen than in adults on unenhanced CT

    d. the spleen has a higher attenuation value than liver on unenhanced CT

    e. the intrahepatic bile ducts are not discernible on unenhanced CT

Q.4.45   In barium examinations of the small bowel

    a. a low residue diet for 24 hours is necessary

    b. placing the patient in the left decubitus position may make it easier to pass a Bilbao Dotter Tube into the duodenum

    c. barium should be diluted to a specific gravity of 3.0 for adults

    d. radiographs should be taken at 80–100 kVp

    e. glucagon may be used to produce small bowel hypertonia

Q.4.46   Contraindications to percutaneous aspiration biopsy of a lung mass under image intensification include

    a. uncorrected bleeding diathesis

    b. lesion invisible on lateral chest radiograph

    c. significantly impaired lung function

    d. known primary malignancy

    e. suspected hydatid disease

For answers see over

Answers

A.4.43 a. T
        b. T
        c. F—The blood flow is very low before day 10; only after day 10 does it increase.
        d. T
        e. T

A.4.44 a. T
        b. F
        c. F
        d. F
        e. T

Daneman A (1987) Pediatric body CT. Springer, Berlin Heidelberg New York.

A.4.45 a. T
        b. T
        c. F—It should be diluted to 1.27 for adults and more dilute for children.
        d. F—They should be taken at 100–120 kVp.
        e. F—Glucagon produces hypotonia.

A.4.46 a. T
        b. T
        c. T
        d. F
        e. T

Q.4.47 **Craniocervical intravenous digital subtraction angiography**

    a. cannot be accomplished successfully following an injection of contrast medium into an antecubital vein

    b. can be achieved with a hand injection of contrast medium in the neonate

    c. uses omnipaque 240 (Iohexol) as a suitable contrast medium

    d. is usually carried out acquiring images at a rate of four images per second

    e. requires contrast medium to be injected at a rate of at least 30 ml/s in the adult

Q.4.48 **Regarding the lower limb vascular studies and anatomy:**

    a. The common femoral vein lies lateral to the femoral artery

    b. In antegrade puncture of the superficial femoral artery internal rotation of the leg may be useful

    c. The profunda femoris artery comes off laterally and posteriorly from the common femoral artery

    d. The groin skin crease is where the subcutaneous tissue is of the least depth with respect to the femoral artery

    e. The deep femoral vein communicates with the popliteal vein

Q.4.49 **In imaging of the biliary tract**

    a. postoperative T-tube cholangiography is unnecessary if tube drainage of bile has ceased

    b. contrast medium injected into hepatic lymphatics at percutaneous transhepatic cholangiography clears very rapidly

    c. the common duct on ultrasound is usually well visualised with the patient in the left anterior oblique position

    d. untreated cholangitis is a contraindication to percutaneous transhepatic cholangiography

    e. ultrasound of the gall bladder is best performed in the fasting patient

For answers see over

Answers

A.4.47 a. F
        b. T
        c. F—This has too low an iodine concentration: "350" or "370" strengths are appropriate.
        d. F—Images are acquired at 1–2 per second.
        e. F—It is injected at 15–20 ml/s.

A.4.48 a. F
        b. F
        c. F
        d. T
        e. F

A.4.49 a. F
        b. F—This is unlike injection into other intrahepatic vessels.
        c. F—The patient should be in the right anterior oblique position.
        d. T—Antibiotic "cover" is essential.
        e. T

Questions

Q.4.50 Regarding cerebral angiography performed with a catheter introduced via the femoral artery:

a. The middle cerebral artery may be opacified following an injection of contrast medium into the vertebral artery
b. The right common carotid artery is usually more difficult to cannulate than the left
c. The catheter tip should be directed posteriorly and laterally to enable its passage from the common to the internal carotid artery in the majority of patients
d. A 6 French gauge Judkins catheter is commonly used for carotid angiography
e. A unilateral carotid artery injection of contrast medium will reliably opacify the major cerebral dural venous sinuses

Q.4.51 The following statements are true:

a. Following intravenous contrast medium, CT can demonstrate the cervical cord at the level of the sixth cervical vertebra
b. With the patient supine, the cerebellar tonsils do not normally descend below the level of the foramen magnum
c. With the latest generation CT scanners, a slice thickness of 4 mm is sufficiently narrow to examine the cervical neural foramina
d. Cervical CT myelography utilising a slice thickness of 4 mm will permit the anterior median fissure of the cervical cord to be discerned
e. A lateral C1–2 puncture for myelography cannot be successfully accomplished with the patient in the supine position

Q.4.52 The position of the cerebellar tonsils may be indicated by

a. vertebral arteriography
b. magnetic resonance imaging
c. uncontrasted axial CT with 1.5 mm sections and coronal reformatting
d. plain film coronal tomography
e. jugular venography

For answers see over

Answers

A.4.50 a. T—Via the posterior communicating arteries.
  b. F
  c. T
  d. F
  e. F—There may be an uneven admixture of opacified and unopacified blood.

A.4.51 a. T
  b. F—Tonsillar descent up to 5 mm below the foramen magnum is permissible.
  c. F—A slice thickness of 1.5–2 mm is necessary.
  d. T
  e. F—The needle is directed to the anterior third of the spinal canal rather than to the posterior third as in the prone position.

A.4.52 a. T—The tonsillar branches of the posterior inferior cerebellar arteries.
  b. T
  c. T
  d. F
  e. F

Q.4.53 With respect to CT scanning:

a. High resolution CT in the axial plane alone is adequate to assess the facial nerve canal

b. Direct coronal CT scanning is the method of choice for the assessment of large tumours of the pituitary region with suprasellar extension

c. The oval and round windows are routinely seen with thin section CT scanning

d. Coronal CT is more useful than axial CT in the assessment of CSF rhinorrhoea after the introduction of intrathecal contrast medium

e. Air CT cisternography should never be done as an outpatient procedure because of the danger of air embolism

Q.4.54 Regarding orbital venography:

a. 2 ml contrast medium is usually sufficient

b. Simultaneous bilateral contrast injection is required for a complete examination

c. The most useful view is the lateral

d. A rubber band around the head at the hairline prevents passage of contrast medium over the scalp

e. An indication for the procedure is suspected cavernous sinus thrombosis

Q.4.55 In radioisotope bone scanning using ^{99m}technetium methylene diphosphonate:

a. In normal subjects, the kidneys eliminate less than 20% of the administered activity

b. In the skeleton, newly formed immature bone concentrates the radiopharmaceutical better than mature bone

c. Uptake in the costal cartilages may be seen as a normal feature

d. Prostatic calcification may be seen as a "hot spot" at the bladder base

e. Due to limited spatial resolution, only lesions greater than 2 cm can be seen

For answers see over

Answers

A.4.53 a. F—Examination of the descending portion requires coronal CT.
        b. F—Axial scanning with sagittal reformatting is important to assess the anterior and posterior extent of the tumour. Coronal scanning is ideal for the diagnosis of microadenomas.
        c. T
        d. T
        e. F

A.4.54 a. F—About 10 ml is needed.
        b. F—Unilateral injection is usually adequate.
        c. F
        d. T
        e. T

A.4.55 a. F
        b. T
        c. T
        d. F
        e. F

Questions

Q.4.56 **The following substances have been used to study gastric emptying:**

a. Scrambled egg labelled with technetium-99m sulphur colloid
b. Technetium-99m–diethylenetriamine penta-acetic acid (DTPA) in 500 ml of saline
c. Paté, labelled in vivo by intraperitoneal injection of technetium sulphur colloid
d. Guinness, prepared from malt raised on an artificial soil substrate containing sodium pertechnetate
e. Sodium pertechnetate given by intravenous injection

Q.4.57 **In myocardial imaging**

a. thallium uptake is significantly inhibited by digoxin
b. technetium-labelled isonitriles are useful imaging agents
c. technetium-labelled pyrophosphate is taken up by healthy myocardium
d. thallium imaging is best commenced 30 minutes after injection, to allow time for pulmonary clearance
e. a multi-pinhole collimeter can be used to obtain tomographic thallium images

Q.4.58 **A recognised complication of**

a. gastrografin enema in meconium ileus is pulmonary oedema
b. lower limb venography is pulmonary embolism
c. pancreatic arteriography for islet cell tumours is profound hypoglycaemia
d. barium enema is infective endocarditis
e. myelography is non-bacterial meningitis

Q.4.59 **The following will normally show enhancement on T1 weighted images following intravenous gadolinium diethylenetriamine penta-acetic acid (DTPA) administration:**

a. Grey matter
b. The choroid plexus
c. The pituitary stalk
d. The external ocular muscles
e. The optic chiasm

For answers see over

Answers

A.4.56 a. T
       b. T
       c. T
       d. F
       e. F

A.4.57 a. F
       b. T
       c. F
       d. F
       e. T

A.4.58 a. F—Decreased circulating blood volume is the fear.
       b. T
       c. F—Although a dextrose infusion would be wise.
       d. T
       e. T

A.4.59 a. F
       b. T
       c. T
       d. F
       e. F

Huk WJ, Gademann G, Friedmann G (1990) MRI of central nervous system diseases. Springer, Berlin Heidelberg New York.

Q.4.60   Flumazenil (Anexate)

    a. is a specific benzodiazepine antagonist
    b. can be administered orally
    c. has a duration of action longer than any of the benzodiaze-
       pines
    d. must not be used in patients with ischaemic heart disease
    e. since it is metabolised primarily by the liver, should be used
       with caution in those with hepatic insufficiency

For answers see over

Answers

A.4.60 a. T
         b. F
         c. F
         d. F
         e. T

Examination 5

Questions

Q.5.1 The decay of a radionuclide by k-electron capture leads to the emission of

    a. alpha-particles
    b. positrons
    c. protons
    d. characteristic x-rays
    e. bremsstrahlung

Q.5.2 The photoelectric effect

    a. is an interaction between a photon and a "free" electron
    b. occurs more frequently as the photon energy increases
    c. is largely responsible for the absorption of x-ray energy by tungstate or rare-earth screens
    d. occurs less frequently in soft tissue than bone
    e. is accompanied by the emission of characteristic radiation

Q.5.3 Ionisation in air or air equivalent materials is commonly used as a measure of the quantity of radiation because

    a. air has a similar atomic number to muscle tissue
    b. the composition of air is the same everywhere
    c. free air chambers are simple to use and are very portable
    d. the energy required to ionise air is similar to x-ray photon energies
    e. ionisation currents are generally of the order of amps

Q.5.4 Scattered radiation reaching the film

    a. causes an overall increase in film density
    b. is always less in energy than the primary beam
    c. can be greater in intensity than the primary photons reaching the film
    d. is removed very effectively by a grid with a grid ratio of 8
    e. is proportionately greater at 100 kV than at 60 kV

For answers see over

Answers

A.5.1 a. F
b. F
c. F
d. T
e. F

A.5.2 a. F—It is an interaction between a photon and a bound electron.
b. F—It depends on E^{-3}.
c. T—Screens are made of high atomic number (Z) materials and the interaction depends upon Z^3.
d. T
e. T

A.5.3 a. T—Both have effective atomic numbers close to 7.64.
b. T
c. F—Free air chambers are national standards.
d. F—On average it takes only 34 eV to form an ion pair in air.
e. F—Depends on the volume of air that is contributing to the current but usually the currents are of the order of pico- or microamps.

A.5.4 a. T
b. T—Compton scattering always reduces photon energy and coherent scattering never contributes a significant effect.
c. T
d. T—Grid ratios between 5 and 12 are usual.
e. T—Although less scatter is produced at the higher kV it has a greater chance of reaching the film due to its higher energy.

Q.5.5   X-ray film emulsion

a. is usually about 20 μm thick
b. is applied to both sides of an acetate base to improve resolution
c. records the latent image by converting silver halide grains into metallic silver
d. has a phosphor density of about 1 mg/cm^3 if the film is to be used with intensifying screens
e. contains a dye to prevent cross-over

Q.5.6   The following contribute to film fog formation:

a. The temperature of the developer
b. The use of a moving grid rather than a fixed grid
c. The latent image
d. Storage of film at 30°C
e. The failure of the reciprocity law when using intensifying screens

Q.5.7   In the use of fluorescent screens in medical radiology

a. the spatial resolution of the image is independent of screen thickness
b. the screen phosphor should have negligible after-glow
c. the screen phosphor should have a high atomic number
d. the screen phosphor produces light whose wavelength depends on the x-ray energy
e. the screen efficiency depends on the density of the phosphor used

Q.5.8   Low ratio grids

a. are easier to manufacture than those of higher ratios
b. result in lower patient doses than those with high ratios
c. can be made by increasing the width of the interspace material
d. are less likely to produce grid cut-off
e. absorb less primary radiation

For answers see over

Answers

A.5.5   a. T—Each emulsion layer is approximately 20 μm thick.

       b. F—Dual emulsion layers improve efficiency but worsen resolution.

       c. F—Development converts grains into metallic silver; exposure produces the latent image as a small speck of silver (maybe only four atoms) within the grain.

       d. F—Film emulsions do not contain phosphors.

       e. F—The acetate base contains the dye.

A.5.6   a. T

       b. F—Fog is unrelated to grid performance.

       c. F—The latent image is formed by exposure to radiation, fog is present without exposure.

       d. T—30 °C is above the recommended storage temperature.

       e. F—Fog is present with or without screens.

A.5.7   a. F—Thicker screens give poorer resolution.

       b. T—Significant after-glow means the screen cannot respond rapidly to changes in intensity and thus is unsuitable.

       c. T—High atomic number means high probability of interaction and thus higher efficiency.

       d. F—Colour fluoroscopy is not available.

       e. T—High density means high probability of interaction and thus higher efficiency.

A.5.8   a. T

       b. T—Lower ratios remove less primary radiation thus less radiation is required.

       c. T—Grid ratio is (height of lead strip)/(interspace width); thus if height is kept constant increasing interspace lowers the ratio.

       d. T

       e. T

Q.5.9   A radiation film badge

    a. must be worn by anybody who might come into contact with ionising radiation

    b. has an accuracy of better than 1%

    c. can give an estimate of both type and quantity of radiation that somebody has been exposed to

    d. should be worn under a lead apron

    e. contains filters, radiation film and intensifying screens

Q.5.10   Regarding testing the kV of a generator:

    a. Weekly tests are required since the kV is generally very unstable

    b. A penetrameter is a test tool that allows the kVp to be estimated to within 3 kV

    c. A kV test tool will only work correctly if the kV is beyond 70 kVp so that the characteristic lines of tungsten have been produced

    d. The kV meter on the x-ray generator can be used to check the kV as it is a direct reading of the generating potential

    e. An aluminium step wedge can be used to make a crude estimate of kV

Q.5.11   Regarding tomography quality control:

    a. The depth of cut is estimated from the width of the image of an exposed slit

    b. Tube motion is checked by exposing a lead disc with a small hole in it, with the disc position at the level of the cut

    c. Uniformity of exposure is checked by exposing a lead disc with a small hole in it, with the disc positioned above or below the level of the cut

    d. Spatial resolution checks cannot be made due to the motion of the tube causing blurring

    e. Noise levels and detectability should be about 0.5% in a linear tomography unit

For answers see over

Answers

A.5.9 a. F—Film badges only need to be worn by persons likely to exceed 3/10 of the maximum permissible dose.

b. F— ± 10% accuracy is probably the best obtainable.

c. T—The optical density gives the quantity of radiation; the comparison between optical densities under all filters gives the type of radiation.

d. T—Recent practice has suggested under the apron or attached to the collar.

e. F—A film badge does not contain intensifying screens.

A.5.10 a. F—kV does not change rapidly and six-monthly tests are more usual.

b. T—Accuracy of the penetrameter depends on its calibration but the precision of the result should be within 3 kV.

c. F—It will test any kV within a reasonable range and is most sensitive to the continuous sprectrum rather than the characteristic lines.

d. F—The kV meter is an indirect reading of the potential.

e. T—The penetration under each step will depend on the kV and thus a crude estimate can be made.

A.5.11 a. F—Depth of cut is estimated using an inclined plane passing through the cut; the linear extent of the image can be related to the depth of cut provided the angle of inclination is known.

b. F—The disc is positioned above or below the level of the cut.

c. T—Both tube motion and uniformity of exposure can be estimated using this method.

d. F—The spatial resolution at the level of the cut can be estimated.

e. F—Noise and detectability will be larger than 0.5%.

Questions

Q.5.12   A reject analysis

a. is a technique for analysing the performance of the film processor
b. is a technique for analysing the performance of x-ray equipment before purchase so that poor equipment can be rejected
c. is a process used to reject poor quality film prior to exposure
d. analyses the reasons why a radiograph is rejected
e. helps in the analysis of all components in the imaging process

Q.5.13   The spatial resolution obtained with a gamma camera

a. depends on the distance from the collimator face to the organ to be imaged
b. depends on the gamma ray energy of the isotope
c. depends on the time taken to scan the source
d. depends on the count rate at which the source is imaged
e. can be improved by increasing the septal length of the collimator

Q.5.14   When a given activity of a radionuclide is administered to a patient for a diagnostic test the radiation dose received by the patient

a. depends on the decay scheme of the isotope
b. depends on the decay constant of the isotope
c. is proportional to the size of the patient
d. is independent of the biological half-life
e. depends on the pharmaceutical to which the isotope is attached

Q.5.15   For safe handling of radioactive solutions administered to patients

a. film badges should be regularly used to monitor contamination
b. lead aprons should be worn
c. lead syringe holders should be used
d. any spill should be mopped up immediately
e. low-activity solutions may be pipetted by mouth

For answers see over

Answers

A.5.12
a. F—It considers more than just the processor (see answers d and e).
b. F—See answers d and e.
c. F—See answers d and e.
d. T—This is the definition of a reject analysis.
e. T—All components contribute to reasons why films are rejected.

A.5.13
a. T—The opening angle of the collimator holes mean that objects further away will be imaged with poorer resolution.
b. T—The collimator design will alter and usually high energy sources give poorer resolution.
c. F—Resolution is a geometrical function of the gamma camera and is unaltered by imaging time.
d. F—Resolution is a geometrical function of the gamma camera, provided count rate is within the camera specification.
e. T—The spatial resolution is proportional to l/d where l is the length of the septa and d is hole diameter.

A.5.14
a. T—The daughter products of the original decay will affect the final dose.
b. T—Isotopes with short half-lives will give lower doses in general as the activity is reduced more quickly.
c. F—Dose is energy imparted per unit mass.
d. F—Biological half life is an indication of the rate of removal of the isotope from the system.
e. T—The pharmaceutical determines the site to which the isotope goes and thus the rate of removal of the activity.

A.5.15
a. F—Film badges are not sensitive enough and do not give an immediate read out.
b. F—Isotope energies are usually too high for "conventional" lead aprons to be of any use.
c. T—Finger doses can be considerably reduced by an easy-to-use lead syringe holder.
d. T—The surface should be monitored with a contamination monitor before and after mopping up.
e. F—No activity should be given the chance of being ingested.

Q.5.16 Regarding CT image display:

a. Small window widths will make the image appear more noisy

b. Brain tissue should be displayed with a window width of approximately 80 HU and at a level of −400 HU

c. The noise on a brain scan image from a well adjusted scanner should be less than 0.5%

d. It is not possible to measure the modulation transfer function (MTF) of a CT scanner because the image is made up of pixels

e. The partial volume effect generally makes high contrast objects appear larger

Q.5.17 The reconstruction filter used in CT scanning

a. improves the quality of the x-ray beam

b. is usually changed according to the part of the body being scanned

c. can usually be changed to improve the detection of low contrast objects or the spatial resolution in fine bony structures

d. is usually 3–5 mm of copper

e. is only used when the data are noisy

Q.5.18 The length of ultrasound pulses is reduced to an absolute minimum so that

a. lateral resolution is improved

b. axial resolution is improved

c. high intensity pulses are produced

d. scattering is reduced

e. penetration is improved

For answers see over

Answers

A.5.16 a. T—Each level of grey in the image has a more restricted range of CT values associated with it and thus variations due to noise become more obvious.
      b. F—At these settings the image would disappear!
      c. T—0.5% or less is the expected noise level.
      d. F—MTF values are often quoted for CT systems although special procedures are required to measure them.
      e. T—Partial volume effects elevate CT values in pixels surrounding a high contrast object.

A.5.17 a. F—The reconstruction filter is used in the mathematics of image reconstruction, it has no effect on the radiation beam.
      b. T—Scans involving large quantities of bone tissue usually use different reconstruction filters than when the abdomen is scanned.
      c. T—"Sharp" filters improve spatial resolution, "soft" filters improve low contrast detectability.
      d. F—See answer a.
      e. F—A reconstruction filter of some sort is always used.

A.5.18 a. F—It is unaffected (see answer b).
      b. T—This is the basic reason for short pulses (range resolution is improved).
      c. F—The amount of energy is often independent of the pulse duration.
      d. F—Scattering is unaffected by pulse length.
      e. F—Penetration (like scattering) depends on frequency not pulse length.

Q.5.19 **A superconducting magnet used in a magnetic resonance (MR) imager**

a. is very sensitive to changes in the Earth's magnetic field
b. is usually longer in physical size than a resistive magnet used for the same purpose
c. uses both liquid helium and liquid nitrogen
d. must always be switched off after use to avoid the windings becoming hot
e. requires a special superconducting power supply

Q.5.20 **Gradient magnetic fields are required**

a. to be changed for each patient
b. so that the signal from a volume element can be isolated
c. so that the volume element will move along the gradient
d. because the main field is not uniform enough
e. only with resistive magnets

Q.5.21 **In cervical spine radiography**

a. in the right posteroanterior oblique position, i.e. with the patient turning his head to his right, the left-sided exit foramina will be disclosed
b. in the right anteroposterior oblique position, the left-sided exit foramina will be disclosed
c. automography is of value in the examination of the atlan-toaxial articulation
d. oblique views are normally taken with the patient erect
e. the large subject-to-film distance for the lateral view causes more definition loss when a fine focus tube is used than when a broad focus tube is used

Q.5.22 **In orthopantomography of the jaws**

a. the detail is as good as with intra-oral films
b. the temporomandibular joints are visible
c. the relationship of the alveolar bone to the tooth is distorted
d. non-screen cassettes are used
e. most images give vertical as well as horizontal magnification

For answers see over

Answers

A.5.19 a. F—The Earth's magnetic field (if it changed) is very small compared with the main field of the magnet.

        b. T—Mechanical considerations require a solenoid shape for strength and a long solenoid for uniformity of field; resistive magnets use different support systems enabling a more compact form.

        c. T—Both coolants are required to reach superconducting temperatures most economically.

        d. F—They cannot be switched off!

        e. F—These do not exist! No current is drawn once running.

A.5.20 a. F—See answer b.

        b. T—This is the purpose of field gradients.

        c. F—See answer b.

        d. F—Shim fields are used to correct non-uniformity.

        e. F—Localisation of the signal is required with all magnets.

A.5.21 a. T

        b. T

        c. T

        d. T

        e. F

A.5.22 a. F

        b. T

        c. T

        d. F

        e. T

Q.5.23 In pelvimetry

a. the "waste space of Morris" refers to the degree of sacral curvature
b. the true conjugate is the corrected measurement from the sacral promontory to the posterosuperior aspect of the pubis
c. on the supine AP view, the maximal transverse inlet is assumed to lie halfway between the symphysis pubis and the table top
d. measurement of the intertuberous diameter on the outlet view is important as clinical assessment of this is poor
e. vaginal delivery is impossible if the fetal biparietal diameter is greater than the AP outlet diameter

Q.5.24 In the majority of people

a. the superior ophthalmic vein does not communicate with the cavernous sinus
b. the internal jugular vein lies medial to the common carotid artery
c. the inferior thyroid veins drain into the internal jugular veins
d. the left superior intercostal vein runs along the left side of the aortic arch
e. the right adrenal vein drains directly into the inferior vena cava

Q.5.25 During development

a. the urachus forms the median umbilical ligament
b. the obliterated umbilical arteries form the medial umbilical ligaments
c. the direction of blood flow through the ductus arteriosus reverses at birth compared with the fetal state
d. the nucleus pulposus of the intervertebral disc develops from the fetal notochord
e. the ureter develops from primitive nephrogenic tissue and grows downwards to fuse with the bladder in the pelvis

For answers see over

Answers

A.5.23 a. F—It refers to the pubic arch.
        b. T
        c. F—It is one-third of the distance between the pubis and the table.
        d. F
        e. F—Moulding of the fetal skull may allow delivery.

A.5.24 a. F—Hence orbital venography.
        b. F
        c. F—They drain into the innominate veins, usually the left.
        d. T—It may simulate a small mass.
        e. T

A.5.25 a. T
        b. T
        c. T
        d. T
        e. F

Questions

Q.5.26 In the normal chest

a. the right main bronchus is shorter than the left main bronchus

b. the right lower lobe apical segment bronchus arises approximately opposite the origin of the middle lobe bronchus

c. bronchial arteries are visible on a chest radiograph

d. the diameter of the lower lobe arteries is less in the prone position than in the supine position

e. the right pulmonary artery is an anterior relation of the superior vena cava

Q.5.27 Concerning the diaphragm:

a. The aorta passes through a hiatus at T12 level

b. The left crus is longer than the right

c. The left crus is sometimes visible on plain abdominal radiographs

d. The thoracic duct passes through the oesophageal hiatus

e. It rises on sniffing

Q.5.28 In relation to the pancreas

a. the minor pancreatic duct of Santorini drains part of the head of the pancreas

b. the duct of Santorini opens above the greater pancreatic duct directly into the duodenum

c. The posterior aspect of the pancreas is covered with peritoneum

d. The inferior pancreaticoduodenal artery is usually a branch of the gastroduodenal artery

e. The pancreatica magna artery is a branch of the splenic artery

Q.5.29 Regarding the anatomy of the adrenal glands:

a. The adrenals lie outside the fascia of Gerota

b. They receive arterial supply from the phrenic arteries superiorly

c. The left adrenal vein is joined by the inferior phrenic vein

d. The right adrenal vein drains into the inferior vena cava near the hepatic vein

e. The adrenal veins have valves

For answers see over

Answers

A.5.26 a. T
           b. T
           c. F
           d. T
           e. F

A.5.27 a. T
           b. F
           c. T
           d. F
           e. F

A.5.28 a. T
           b. T
           c. F
           d. F
           e. T

A.5.29 a. F
           b. T
           c. T
           d. T
           e. F

Q.5.30 Immediate anterior relations of the abdominal aorta include:

a. Transverse colon
b. Right renal vein
c. The third (transverse) portion of the duodenum
d. Superior mesenteric artery
e. Head of the pancreas

Q.5.31 The following bones articulate with each other by synovial joints:

a. Trapezoid and second metacarpal
b. Manubrium and body of sternum
c. Lateral cuneiform and fifth metatarsal
d. Proximal tibia and head of fibula
e. Malleus and stapes

Q.5.32 Lymphatics from the following drain to the internal iliac nodes:

a. The ovary
b. The prostate gland
c. The seminal vesicles
d. The uterine tubes
e. The uterine body

Q.5.33 The ischiorectal fossa

a. contains the superior rectal vessels
b. contains the pudendal nerve
c. is bounded superolaterally by levator ani
d. is readily identified on axial CT
e. contains the inferior rectal vessels

Q.5.34 The frontal sinuses

a. drain to the superior nasal meatus
b. are normally apparent in radiographs taken in the first year of life
c. form part of the orbital roof
d. are reliably symmetrical
e. are best demonstrated radiologically by an occipitomental projection

For answers see over

Answers

A.5.30 a. F
          b. F
          c. T
          d. T
          e. F

A.5.31 a. T
          b. F—This joint is not synovial.
          c. F
          d. T
          e. F

A.5.32 a. F
          b. T
          c. T
          d. F
          e. F

A.5.33 a. F
          b. T
          c. F—It is bounded superomedially by levator ani.
          d. T
          e. T

A.5.34 a. F—They drain to the middle meatus.
          b. F
          c. T
          d. F
          e. F

Q.5.35 **Concerning the larynx:**

a. The true vocal cords lie superior to the cricothyroid membrane
b. The cricoid cartilage forms a complete ring in transverse section
c. The aryepiglottic folds move apart during swallowing
d. The true vocal cords are abducted during gentle respiration
e. The epiglottis commonly calcifies or ossifies in the adult

Q.5.36 **The following are true statements:**

a. The lacrimal gland is situated in the superomedial part of the orbit
b. A single canaliculus drains to the lacrimal sac at the medial canthus
c. The nasolacrimal duct drains into the inferior meatus of the nose
d. The lacrimal gland is supplied by the ophthalmic artery
e. The lacrimal gland is innervated by the facial nerve through the pterygopalatine ganglion

Q.5.37 **Regarding dental radiology:**

a. Dentine has a radiodensity comparable to compact bone
b. The cementum can be reliably distinguished from the adjacent dentine
c. The normal adult mandible possesses two premolars
d. The lower permanent dentition normally erupts before the upper
e. Teeth are normally borne on the ramus of the mandible

Q.5.38 **The oculomotor nerve**

a. courses along the floor of the cavernous sinus
b. arises from the pons
c. supplies the inferior oblique muscle
d. lies lateral to the posterior communicating artery in the interpenduncular cistern
e. divisions enter the orbit by both superior and inferior orbital fissures

For answers see over

Answers

A.5.35 a. T
      b. T
      c. F—They move together.
      d. T
      e. F—This is unlike other laryngeal cartilages.

A.5.36 a. F—It is in the superolateral part of the orbit.
      b. F—There are two.
      c. T
      d. T
      e. T

A.5.37 a. T
      b. F
      c. F
      d. T
      e. F

A.5.38 a. F
      b. F
      c. T
      d. T
      e. F

Q.5.39 The optic nerve

a. is invested by a dural sheath which it shares with the ophthalmic artery
b. travels in an axial plane which is approximately parallel to the anthropological baseline
c. is appropriately examined with axial CT at a window width of 250 HU
d. may become surrounded by contrast following an intrathecal injection of contrast medium
e. should invariably be examined before and after intravenous contrast administration

Q.5.40 The quadrigeminal cistern

a. is an irregular space well seen in CT and MRI scans
b. contains the posterior choroidal arteries
c. is related to the pons anteriorly
d. is bounded posteriorly by the tenorium and falx
e. contains a large venous confluence

Q.5.41 In CT of the body

a. the thymus is usually visible in adults
b. a vaginal tampon filled with contrast is used in examination of the true pelvis
c. bowel opacification may be obtained using a 10% solution of gastrograffin
d. a left lateral decubitus examination is commonly used to show the head of the pancreas
e. the bladder should be filled for examinations of the true pelvis

For answers see over

Answers

A.5.39 a. T
b. T
c. T
d. T
e. F—Unenhanced CT alone is often sufficient.

Newton TH, Hasso AN, Dillon WP (eds) (1988) Computed tomography of the head and neck (Modern neuroradiology, vol 3). Raven Press, New York.

A.5.40 a. T
b. T
c. F—The quadrigeminal bodies are part of the midbrain.
d. T
e. T

A.5.41 a. T
b. F
c. F
d. F—Right lateral decubitus.
e. T

Q.5.42 Concerning intravenous urography:

   a. The density of the nephrogram is increased in dehydrated subjects

   b. Pyelotubular opacification ("papillary blush") is seen more commonly with low-osmolar than with high-osmolar contrast

   c. Ureteric compression devices should be applied at the level of the umbilicus

   d. Radiographic exposures within the range 90–100 kV are optimal

   e. Non-obstructive ureteric dilation of pregnancy is commonly more marked on the right side

Q.5.43 In the Whitaker test

   a. a catheter is placed in the rectum so that intra-abdominal pressure may be measured

   b. a spinal needle should ideally be placed in a posterior calyx

   c. saline is infused at a rate of 20 ml/min

   d. a second fine-bore needle should be inserted into the collecting system to measure pressure

   e. fluoroscopy may help to show the level of obstruction

Q.5.44 Regarding antenatal ultrasound:

   a. Fetal heart pulsations are first detectable by about 10 weeks gestational age

   b. Placental localisation may be difficult in the first trimester

   c. The gestation sac may be identified after 5 weeks' amenorrhoea

   d. Fetal kidneys cannot be identified before 20 weeks' gestation

   e. The yolk sac appears as a circular transsonic structure in the gestation sac

For answers see over

Answers

A.5.42 a. F
        b. T
        c. F
        d. F—60–80 kV is optimal.
        e. T

A.5.43 a. F
        b. T
        c. F—It is infused at 10 ml/min.
        d. T
        e. T

A.5.44 a. F—They are first detectable at about 6 weeks.
        b. T
        c. T
        d. F—They can be identified from about 14 weeks onwards.
        e. T

Chudleigh P, Pearce JM (1986) Obstetric ultrasound. Churchill Livingstone, Edinburgh.

Q.5.45 Transvaginal ultrasonography

  a. is not as well accepted by patients as abdominal pelvic ultrasound
  b. commonly uses a 5 MHz probe
  c. may be combined with bimanual examination to move pelvic organs close to the probe
  d. gives better visualisation of the ovaries than abdominal ultrasound
  e. is carried out with the patient in the Trendelenberg position with the pelvis raised

Q.5.46 Ultrasonography of the infant brain

  a. replaces CT in many instances
  b. is best performed with a linear array probe
  c. readily demonstrates Sylvian fissures in the normal brain
  d. shows the cavum septum pellucidum in half of neonates at term
  e. shows the parenchyma of the cerebellum as less echogenic than that of the cerebral hemispheres

Q.5.47 In the examination of the oesophagus

  a. the use of Buscopan (hyoscine butylbromide) may obscure visualisation of small varices
  b. a bread–barium swallow is useful for the assessment of narrow oesophageal strictures
  c. rapid sequential swallowing in the prone position is the optimum method for assessing peristalsis
  d. aspiration of barium into the bronchial tree is of no significance
  e. an aberrant right subclavian artery causes an anterior indentation of the barium column

For answers see over

Answers

A.5.45 a. F
       b. F
       c. T
       d. T
       e. F

Timor-Tritsch IE, Rottem S (1988) Transvaginal sonography. Heinemann Medical, London.

A.5.46 a. T
       b. F
       c. T
       d. T
       e. F

A.5.47 a. F
       b. F—It is usually employed to evaluate the functional significance of minor strictures or narrowings.
       c. F—A single bolus is used.
       d. F
       e. F—It causes a posterior indentation.

Questions

Q.5.48 **Regarding radiological reduction of intussusception in infants:**

a. It is contraindicated when signs of peritonitis are present
b. Gastrograffin is the preferred contrast medium
c. Contrast medium is introduced by syringe using hand pressure
d. Opacification of the terminal ileum indicates complete reduction
e. Reduction using saline can be performed under ultrasound guidance

Q.5.49 **During a barium enema examination**

a. radiography at about 60 kv is optimal for double contrast studies
b. perforation occurs more commonly when a catheter with an inflatable cuff is used
c. caudal angulation of the x-ray beam reduces overlapping of sigmoid loops
d. the left anterior oblique projection demonstrates the hepatic flexure well
e. passage of barium into the small bowel is reduced by the patient lying in the prone position

Q.5.50 **Regarding oral cholecystography:**

a. Sodium ioglycamate is commonly used
b. Subsequent uptake of iodine by the thyroid gland is reduced for at least 2 months
c. Oral cholecystographic agents are mainly bound to plasma albumen
d. The oral contrast agents are di-iodinated
e. Oral cholecystographic agents are excreted in the bile by a passive process.

For answers see over

Answers

A.5.48 a. T
        b. F
        c. F
        d. T
        e. T

A.5.49 a. F—This is too low.
        b. T
        c. T
        d. F
        e. T

A.5.50 a. F
        b. T
        c. T
        d. F
        e. F—They are excreted by an active process, in competition with bilirubin.

Q.5.51 In percutaneous transhepatic cholangiography and stent insertion

   a. high density contrast is used
   b. ascites is a contraindication
   c. antibiotic cover is indicated
   d. five passes with a fine needle are permissible as standard practice in a non-dilated system
   e. stent insertion may be complicated by pneumothorax

Q.5.52 Regarding endoscopic retrograde choledochopancreatography:

   a. Contrast medium containing about 300 mg iodine per ml is suitable for pancreatic duct studies
   b. The purpose of intravenous hyoscine *n*-butyl bromide (Buscopan) is to delay emptying of the pancreatic duct
   c. The diameter of the common bile duct is difficult to estimate owing to variable magnification on different views
   d. Prior peptic ulcer surgery may make the procedure impossible
   e. Failure of immediate gall bladder filling with biliary injection of contrast is pathological

Q.5.53 Regarding bronchography:

   a. It is more accurate than CT in the evaluation of bronchiectasis
   b. Dionosil aqueous may be used in a dose of 20 ml per side in adults
   c. Dribbling contrast medium over the back of the patient's tongue is a good technique
   d. The cricothyroid puncture method may result in mediastinitis
   e. Headache occurs as a recognised side-effect

For answers see over

Answers

A.5.51 a. F
    b. T
    c. T
    d. T
    e. T

A.5.52 a. T
    b. F—It facilitates endoscopic cannulation of the ducts.
    c. F—The diameter of the endoscope can be used as a standard.
    d. T
    e. F

A.5.53 a. T
    b. F—The maximum dose should be 12–16 ml per side.
    c. F—It does not allow a selective examination.
    d. T
    e. T

Questions

Q.5.54 **Digital subtraction angiography with selective arterial cannulation (arterial DSA)**

a. as with intravenous DSA, requires an injection of contrast medium prior to the acquisition of subtracted images
b. is inappropriate for carotid angiography following direct cervical arterial puncture
c. is known to have a superior spatial resolution to conventional film-screen angiography
d. is greatly dependent on left ventricular function for the adequate display of peripheral arteries
e. unlike conventional film-screen angiography, permits the accurate measurement of the diameter of an intracranial aneurysm

Q.5.55 **In angiography safety and diagnostic accuracy are enhanced by**

a. using catheters with side holes for selective angiography
b. flushing the catheter with saline if ionic contrast medium is used although non-ionic contrast can safely be left in the catheter between injections
c. ensuring that injection rates in selective catheterisation approximate to the normal flow blood for that vessel
d. ensuring that a "flexible" guide wire exiting from a catheter is more than 1 cm beyond the tip before the properly flexible portion begins
e. ensuring that the stiff portion of a guide wire is in the selected artery before the catheter is advanced

Q.5.56 **Regarding the vertebral arteries:**

a. They give off no cervical branches
b. The right is usually more easily selectively catheterised than the left
c. Cerebral panangiography for a suspected intracranial aneurysm must involve catheterisation of both vertebral arteries
d. The catheter tip for vertebral angiography should ideally be at the level of the body of the second cervical vertebra
e. Blindness is a recognised complication of vertebral angiography

For answers see over

Answers

A.5.54 a. F—It is required after the acquisition of subtracted images.
         b. F
         c. F
         d. F
         e. F

A.5.55 a. T
         b. F
         c. T
         d. T
         e. T

A.5.56 a. F
         b. F
         c. F—Injection of one vertebral artery will frequently be associated with reflux of contrast medium into the other.
         d. F—This is too high.
         e. T

Questions

Q.5.57 **The following radiopharmaceuticals can be used for isotope brain scanning:**

a. Sodium pertechnetate (^{99m}Tc)
b. Technetium-99m-hydroxymethyl propylene amineoxime (HMPAO)
c. Technetium-99m-glucohepatonate
d. Indium-111 oxine
e. Stannous (^{112}Sn) chloride

Q.5.58 **The following statements are true:**

a. Labelled monoclonal antibodies can be used in vivo to demonstrate tumours
b. Labelled nanocolloid can be injected subcutaneously to demonstrate lymph nodes
c. Technetium-99m in particle form can be injected intra-articularly to demonstrate synovitis
d. Sodium pertechnetate ^{99m}Tc is the most suitable radiopharmaceutical for demonstrating a lingual thyroid
e. Krypton-81m in solution can be used for studying myocardial perfusion

Q.5.59 **The following preclude a patient from undergoing a cranial MRI investigation:**

a. The need for a general anaesthetic
b. Temporal lobe epilepsy
c. The presence of a cardiac pacemaker
d. The presence of any type of intracranial aneurysm clip
e. The presence of a prosthetic hip implant

Q.5.60 **Intravenous gadolinium DTPA**

a. results in a high signal return from the cerebral arteries on a T1 weighted image
b. causes enhancement of the maxillary antral mucosa as a normal finding on a T1 weighted image
c. is administered at a recommended intravenous dose of 0.5 mmol/kg body weight
d. is excreted predominantly in the bile
e. results in the patient experiencing a feeling of generalised warmth 30 s after administration

For answers see over

Answers

A.5.57 a. T
        b. T
        c. T
        d. F
        e. F

A.5.58 a. T
        b. T
        c. F
        d. F
        e. T

A.5.59 a. F
        b. F
        c. T
        d. F
        e. F

Huk WJ, Gademann G, Friedmann G (1990) MRI of central nervous system diseases. Springer, Berlin Heidelberg New York.

A.5.60 a. F—Rapidly flowing blood results in a signal void.
        b. T
        c. F—A dose of 0.1 mmol/kg is recommended.
        d. F
        e. F